LABORATORY TESTS
in common use

laboratory tests

IN COMMON USE

SOLOMON GARB, M.D., F.A.C.P.
Scientific Director, American Medical
Center at Denver
Associate Clinical Professor of Medicine,
University of Colorado Medical School

SIXTH EDITION

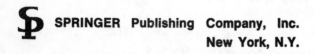

SPRINGER Publishing Company, Inc.
New York, N.Y.

Copyright © 1976

Springer Publishing Company, Inc.
200 Park Avenue South
New York, N.Y. 10003

76 77 78 79 80 / 10 9 8 7 6 5 4 3 2

Sixth edition, January 1976
Fifth edition, September 1971
Fourth edition, November 1966
Third edition, September 1963
Second edition, September 1959
First edition, April 1956

Library of Congress Catalog Card Number: 73-161127

Standard Book Numbers: 0-8261-0188-7 (cloth edition)
                        0-8261-0187-9 (paper edition)

Printed in U.S.A.

Preface to Sixth Edition

This edition continues the format of previous editions. The listings of drugs and foods that may interfere with laboratory tests have been expanded. Unfortunately, our knowledge of such interferences is still limited, and there are probably many more situations in which drugs and foods can result in spurious laboratory test results.

Several obsolete tests have been deleted and approximately thirty new tests have been added to bring the edition up to date. Laboratory tests have become increasingly complex, and automated methods are widespread. No attempt has been made to describe the laboratory procedures fully. There are many excellent books that do so.

I want to express my appreciation to Vincent Lagerborg, M.D., Ph.D., Chief of Pathology at American Medical Center at Denver, and to Jerry Aikawa, M.D., Professor of Pathology and Director of Laboratories at the University of Colorado Medical School, for their review of the manuscript and many helpful suggestions. However, I am solely responsible for any errors or omissions to be found. I am also grateful to Ms. Mary L. Wickens and Ms. Sue Strakey for their efficient secretarial help.

Contents

1

Introduction

Laboratory tests aid in the diagnosis and management of various disorders. Tests included in this book are, for the most part, those in relatively common use. In a few cases, tests that are not yet in common use are described if it seems likely that they will be in common use in the near future.

A test may be ordered by a physician to confirm his suspicion or impression, or it may be performed routinely on most or all patients. Routine tests are carried out because the disorders they demonstrate are relatively common and the tests themselves relatively easy to perform. An example of this sort of test is the determination of blood hemoglobin concentration. A substantial proportion of the population has anemia, so that this test, performed on 100 patients with complaints not related to the blood, will reveal several who would benefit from antianemia therapy. Hemoglobin, serology, and urinalysis examinations are performed routinely on most patients. Many physicians and hospitals also include a blood count, test of the feces for blood, chest x-ray, and an electrocardiogram.

Some tests have no significance other than to indicate the diagnosis. An example of this is the glucose tolerance test. Should the result of such a test indicate the presence of diabetes, the test is of no further use in regulating treatment. Many tests, however, can be useful in following the course of the disease or in adjusting therapy. An example of the latter is the test for prothrombin time. In treatment with dicumarol and similar drugs, tests for prothrombin time are performed daily to aid in prescribing the correct dose of dicumarol for the current day.

In some institutions a single laboratory performs all the tests; in others there may be several laboratories, one performing bacteriological tests, another chemical tests, and so on.

The origin of the test material does not always correspond to the organ or system being examined. A test may be performed on urine to obtain information on liver function. Since, in the following chapters, most tests are arranged according to the type of specimen examined (i.e., blood, urine, etc.), Tables 1–9 are included as a supplement that groups the tests according to the organ or system whose functions are being tested.

It should be noted that many of the tests are useful in diagnosing diseases of more than one organ or system. This, of course, is a natural consequence of the interrelationship between the various organs and systems of the body. In many cases, therefore, the interpretation of the results of these tests by the physician is not simply a matter of routine but involves careful integration with history and physical findings.

In some cases the relationship of a laboratory test to the pathological physiology of a disease is clear. For example, since the kidney excretes urea, it might be predicted that in advanced kidney disease the blood urea levels will be elevated. On the other hand, the exact relationship of some laboratory tests to the pathological physiology of disease is not known. An example of this is the thymol turbidity test for liver function. In these cases it has been found empirically that the tests are usually positive in certain types of disorders. There are theories that attempt to correlate the test results with the disease process, but since they are unproven, and in most cases highly complex, they are not discussed in this book. Other tests, such as the determination of the sedimentation rate, are so nonspecific that they do not point to any particular group of diseases, but only indicate that there is some disorder.

Drugs　In evaluating laboratory tests, it is always advisable to consider the drugs that a patient is receiving. In a number of cases, these drugs can affect the test results and produce an erroneous diagnosis. As more and more drugs are developed, this problem will increase in complexity. New drugs are being developed so rapidly at present that even an up-to-date book may not be a complete enough guide to the ways in which drugs can interfere with laboratory tests. Furthermore, the physician in charge of the patient is seldom aware of technical details of laboratory procedures and the ways in which drugs can interfere with them. On the other hand, the clinical pathologist in charge of the laboratory, who does have this information, may not know which drugs have been administered to the patient. The nurse is in a position to help solve this problem. In most hospitals, the laboratory slip, which is sent from the ward to the laboratory along with the specimen, has a space for a brief clinical summary or impression. It is suggested that the nurse include therein a list of all the drugs the patient has received in the past 72 hours. Perhaps, in the future, these laboratory slips will include a special space for listing all drugs being administered to the patient.

In the discussion of each test described in this book, a special section lists the known drugs, foods, and procedures that have been reported to interfere with or give erroneous results in laboratory tests. Although every effort has been made to include important published information on interference with laboratory test results, it must be assumed that the information listed is incomplete.

We do not know in every case whether the drugs listed are likely to interfere with a test occasionally, usually, or all the time. Accordingly, it may be quite proper for a physician to order a laboratory test even though he knows that a potentially interfering drug is being administered, provided his interpretation of the results considers the possible effects of interference. On the other hand, it is certainly preferable to do the tests in the absence of potentially interfering materials.

There are several mechanisms whereby laboratory results may be changed by interfering materials. In some cases, there is an effect on the laboratory procedure, resulting in an incorrect measurement. For example, the test for bilirubin is based on the color of the serum. If the patient has taken a drug or a food that gives a yellowish color to the serum, the test reading will be high, even though the actual bilirubin level may be normal.

In other cases, a food, medication, or test material may contribute increased amounts of a particular substance to body fluids. The actual test reading may be perfectly correct and accurate, but it may still be misleading if the role of the additional substance is not recognized. For example, in possible cases of hypothyroidism, a low protein-bound iodine is an important diagnostic point. Many drugs (Table 22), including over-the-counter remedies, contain iodine, and may produce an elevation of the protein-bound iodine. If a patient has taken one of these drugs and has an elevated protein-bound iodine level as a result, the physician may be misled in his diagnosis unless he is aware of the possible effects of the drug on the test results.

In other situations, drugs may confuse the diagnosis because of mild to moderate toxic effects on some organs. If a patient has obscure symptoms that the physician is trying to diagnose, several tests of liver function may be ordered, including transaminase levels (SGOT). Many drugs can elevate SGOT levels, probably because of slight toxic effects on the liver. If the patient has taken one of these drugs and the physician is not aware of it, or of the possible relationship to test results, he could mistakenly conclude that the probable diagnosis is early liver disease when, in actuality, an entirely different condition might be involved.

It must be borne in mind that the information in this book is a summary of the available knowledge of the subject. The descriptions of the laboratory tests themselves are abbreviated as much as possible. A laboratory test described in 2 or 3 lines here might require 2 or 3 pages of description in order to enable the reader to understand it fully and to perform it. For a thorough understanding of the laboratory procedures, a standard book on laboratory methods should be consulted.

The vast majority of clinical conditions in which laboratory tests aid in diagnosis will be covered by the tests in this book. However, in some cases in which the diagnosis is still obscure after the usual test results are available, the physician may need to employ a group of tests or some additional, less common tests. This occurs mainly with the liver diseases and with some chronic disorders of connective tissue. On the basis of clinical experience, tables have been devised to help the physician (usually a consultant) use a series of test results to arrive at a correct diagnosis of an obscure ailment. Material of this sort is beyond the scope of this book, and the reader who wishes to have such information is directed to the more comprehensive texts and the original clinical studies.

As additional aids Chapters 8 and 9 and Tables 10–27 are included.

Part One

Tests According to Type
of Specimen Employed

2

Microbiological Tests

Materials collected for bacteriological examination fall into two groups: (1) cultures made at the bedside, and (2) specimens to be cultured in the laboratory.

A *culture* consists of material inoculated directly into a culture medium. In most hospitals only nose and throat secretions and venous blood are put into culture media at the bedside. The culture should be placed in an incubator at once, so that the bacteria may grow.

A *specimen* consists of material that will be cultured in the laboratory. All bacteriological specimens, other than spinal fluid, are kept in the bacteriological refrigerator to preserve the organisms. Spinal fluid may contain organisms that are sensitive to cold and is therefore placed in a bacteriological incubator.

In handling specimens and cultures for bacteriological examinations, it is at all times essential to keep in mind the possible danger of spreading infectious agents. All persons handling bacteriological material must know the necessary protective procedures. It is also important that the specimens reach the laboratory in a condition suitable for culture. Accordingly, the following precautions must be observed:

1. Use standard equipment. Do not substitute other containers for those designated by the laboratory.
2. Do not use cracked or broken containers.
3. Use only the regulation plugs to stopper tubes and bottles. Do not substitute gauze, paper, ordinary cotton, or other materials.
4. Do not use applicators that are broken or in any way contaminated.
5. Use only one applicator per tube.

6. Do not use Petri dishes for fluid specimens or those which ooze fluids, including blood.
7. Remove plugs from containers gently, with a twisting motion; do not pull straight out.
8. Discard any plug that comes in contact with an unsterile surface.
9. Do not fill containers more than half full.
10. Do not allow plugs to become wet, either from the specimen or from other sources. Wet plugs may contaminate personnel handling them and may also contaminate the specimen.
11. Do not spill any material on the outside of containers, plugs, boxes, tables, etc. If such material is spilled accidentally, call the bacteriology laboratory to find out how best to destroy the infectious agent. Ordinary soap and water may not be adequate. Do not allow anyone to come near the spilled material.
12. Make sure that plugs are firmly in place when the procedure is completed.
13. Plugs should be rotated clockwise.
14. Specimens and cultures should be carried in an upright position, and should not be shaken.
15. After collection, the specimen should be sent to the laboratory at once.
16. Certain organisms, such as the gonococcus and the Pertussis and Brucella groups, need freshly prepared culture media. Therefore, if the presence of those organisms is suspected, the laboratory must be notified at least an hour before the specimen is to be collected.

Agglutination Tests

The blood is tested for substances made by the body to neutralize a particular invading organism. These substances, known as agglutinins, cause such microorganisms to clump together. When specific agglutinins are present, they indicate that the body has been exposed to the microorganism in question and has developed some immunity to it. This procedure can be used with a large variety of microorganisms. However, only three groups are usually tested for in most laboratories in this country. They are:

1. The Brucella, or undulant fever, group of bacteria.
2. The typhoid and paratyphoid group of bacteria. The Widal test is used.
3. Rickettsia. This agglutination reaction differs from the others in that the organism which is agglutinated is not the Rickettsia itself but a bacterium, Proteus OX19, which for some unknown reason is agglutinated by the antirickettsial agglutinins. The test used is also known as the Weil-Felix test.

There is an important consideration in judging the results of these tests. A positive test indicates only that the patient harbored the microorganism *at some time;* it does not necessarily indicate that the organism is still present. A patient who had the suspected disease years previously may still have a positive agglutination reaction.

Food and drink restrictions None.

Procedure for collecting specimen Collect 5 ml of *venous* blood in a collecting tube with a red stopper. The tests are performed on the serum. The quantity is sufficient for all three agglutination tests. Particular care must be exercised to prevent spilling blood on the outside of the test tube since blood may contain virulent organisms.

Laboratory procedure The laboratory adds serial dilutions of the patient's serum to suspensions of either live or killed bacteria. Observations are then made, sometimes with and sometimes without a microscope, to see whether clumping has occurred and to determine the range of dilutions within which the agglutination takes place. The dilutions ordinarily used range up to 1:1024. When live bacteria are used, they remain virulent when agglutinated and must be disposed of carefully.

Possible interfering materials and conditions If the patient has received antibiotics or chemotherapy (such as sulfonamides) there may be a false negative reaction.

Normal range Normal people sometimes have small amounts of agglutinin in their blood. Accordingly, the lowest concentration of the serum at which agglutination takes place is important. In the Widal test for typhoid fever, a positive agglutination at a concentration of 1:160 and up is required for a definite diagnosis. Separate measurements of O, H, and V antigens may be made.

In the diagnosis of brucellosis by agglutination, a positive response at serum dilution of 1:50 or over is required, depending on the results of the skin test.

In the Weil-Felix test for rickettsial disease, agglutination must take place at serum dilutions of 1:160 or more for the test to be positive.

If there is doubt as to whether a positive agglutination test comes from a current infection or an earlier one, repeated tests may be performed at intervals of 3 to 5 days. Agglutination in progressively higher dilutions of serum strongly suggests a current infection.

Antibiotic Sensitivity Test

It is sometimes important to know which antibiotic is most effective against a particular strain of bacteria causing a patient's illness. This can usually be determined in the laboratory, using the disc or tube dilution methods. Since there are many variables that determine the effectiveness of antibiotics, these tests are only suggestive.

Food and drink restrictions   None.

Procedure for collecting specimen   The same as for corresponding cultures.

If both antibiotic sensitivity and blood culture tests are ordered at the same time, it may be possible to do both on the blood culture material. However, this will vary according to the system used in a particular laboratory, and the laboratory should be consulted first.

Laboratory procedure   The ability of various antibiotics to stop or slow the multiplication of bacteria is measured. Several methods may be used, the most common of which is the disc method, which involves placing small discs of filter paper containing an antibiotic on a Petri dish streaked with a culture of the bacteria. The width of the zone of growth inhibition around the disc determines the sensitivity of the organism to the antibiotic. In the tube dilution method, the bacteria are cultured in a series of tubes containing known concentrations of an antibiotic. The lowest concentration that completely inhibits multiplication of the bacteria determines the sensitivity of the organism.

Possible interfering materials and conditions   If the patient has received antibiotic or chemotherapy (such as sulfonamides) there may be a false negative reaction.

Blood Culture

Many varieties of bacteria produce bacteremia or bloodstream infections. Frequently, a precise identification of the offending microorganism is necessary to enable the physician to select the appropriate antibiotic. Some types of bacteria do not survive changes in temperature or prolonged standing in the absence of special culture media, so that it is impractical to send a specimen of venous blood to be cultured. The procedure, therefore, is carried out at the bedside.

Food and drink restrictions   None.

Procedure for collecting specimen   Several different procedures are available. The patient's skin must be properly prepared with an effective antiseptic. Either benzalkonium chloride or iodine followed by alcohol may be used. Newer methods of obtaining blood cultures are based on the use of prepared blood culture media in special vacuum tubes. The amount of blood required varies with different laboratories. Collect the specified amount of *venous* blood in a collecting tube with a yellow stopper.

Laboratory procedure   Laboratory personnel will observe the cultures at regular intervals. If bacteriological growth appears, they will endeavor to identify the organism by direct smears. Frequently they will have to make one or more subcultures for positive identification. Final reports may therefore be delayed as long as 10 days. Usually, however, preliminary reports on blood cultures are available after 36 hours.

Possible interfering materials and conditions   If the patient has received antibiotics or chemotherapy (such as sulfonamides) there may be a false negative reaction.

Normal range   Normal blood should be sterile. Any microorganism found in the blood culture is either a contaminant from an imperfect procedure or an indication of a pathological condition.

Dark-field Examination

This bacteriological examination is usually done to determine whether the Treponema of syphilis is present. The test is performed on fluid that oozes out of lesions of skin or mucous membranes, not on blood. This special type of examination is needed because the Treponema is too thin to be seen by ordinary microscopic techniques, but can be seen by reflected light in a dark field.

Food and drink restrictions None.

Procedure for collecting specimen The specimen is collected by the person (usually a bacteriologist or pathologist) doing the examination. In most institutions the patient is brought to the laboratory for this examination.

Precaution Material from a dark-field positive lesion is highly infectious. All personnel who may come in contact with it should be protected.

Laboratory procedure The material is examined in a dark field for the Treponema pallidum. When an oral lesion is under examination, careful observation is needed to distinguish the Treponema pallidum from similar forms that are normally found in the mouth and that do not cause disease.

Possible interfering materials and conditions If the patient has received antibiotics there may be a false negative reaction.

Normal range Normally no Treponema pallidum will be seen.

Fluorescent Antibody

This is a rapid test for the identification of microorganisms. It is usually used to determine the type of organism involved in an infection so that the most appropriate antibiotic can be chosen at once. This procedure also can be used to identify particular microorganisms in a mixture of many types. It can identify bacteria, protozoa, viruses, and proteins. In medicolegal applications, a similar technique can be used to identify the species origin of minute blood stains. In epidemiological studies, a similar technique can determine the species of animal upon which a mosquito has last fed. There are also Civil Defense aspects to this test. Since it can identify organisms within a matter of minutes, it could be used in suspected biological warfare attacks to determine which organisms are being spread.

A recent development is the fluorescent treponemal antibody test. In this test, the ability of a patient's serum to coat treponemes is measured. Although this is probably the most specific and sensitive of all the serologic tests for syphilis, it requires special techniques and training and is not yet performed in most hospitals. However, if advisable, the patient's serum may be sent for testing to an institution that does perform this procedure, such as a state public health laboratory.

Food and drink restrictions   None.

Procedure for collecting specimen   Specimens are collected in a sterile, clean, disposable container and sent to the laboratory at once. This test may be done on almost any type of body fluid. It is advisable to indicate to the laboratory which microorganisms are suspected.

Laboratory procedure   Specific antisera, conjugated with a fluorescent material (fluorescein isothiocyanate), which may be obtained from several commercial sources, are used. The specimen to be examined is fixed to a slide and fluorescent antiserum layered over it. After a few minutes, the excess antiserum is washed off and the slide examined by ultraviolet light with a special microscope. If any of the fluorescein remains, it will glow in the ultraviolet light. When the test is properly performed, the fluorescence will be seen only when the antibody has combined with the proper antigen. For example, if it is suspected that there are typhoid bacilli in a specimen, the laboratory will place fluorescein conjugated antityphoid antiserum on the slide. After washing, the antityphoid antiserum would remain and fluoresce only if typhoid bacilli were present in the specimen.

Possible interfering materials and conditions   If the patient has received antibiotics or chemotherapy (such as sulfonamides) there may be a false negative reaction.

Normal range   This depends on the type of specimen being examined.

Fluorescent Treponemal Antibody Absorption (FTA-ABS)

This is a test for syphilis, the most sensitive currently known. It is used when other tests suggest syphilis, but when a false positive reaction must be ruled out.

Food and drink restrictions   None reported.

Procedure for collecting specimen   Collect 5 ml of *venous* blood in a collecting tube with a red stopper.

Laboratory procedure   The procedure is much more complex than that required for most serological tests for syphilis, and not all laboratories can perform it. In essence, the patient's serum is allowed to react with stored treponemes on a slide. Then, a fluorescein-labeled antihuman globulin is added, and the slide examined with a fluorescent microscope.

Possible interfering materials and conditions   In some cases of lupus erythematosus, a partial fluorescence consisting of a "beaded" pattern may be seen.

Normal range   Normally, this test is negative.

Miscellaneous Fluid Cultures

Various body cavities sometimes fill with fluid that may contain bacteria. The pleural, peritoneal, and pericardial cavities are most commonly involved.

Food and drink restrictions   None.

Procedure for collecting specimen   The physician removes the specimen and places it in a sterile tube, using aseptic technique.

Laboratory procedure   Essentially the same as in blood culture test.

Possible interfering materials and conditions   If the patient has received antibiotics or chemotherapy (such as sulfonamides) there may be a false negative reaction.

Normal range   Normally these body cavities are sterile. Therefore, any bacteria found in the culture are either pathogens or contaminants resulting from an imperfect collection procedure.

Nose and Throat Culture

It is frequently useful for the physician to know which bacteria are present in the nose and throat. This information is obtained by means of a nose and throat culture.

Food and drink restrictions   None.

Procedure for collecting specimen   The physician collects the specimen on a sterile cotton swab. The swab is suspended in a sterile culture tube containing 2 ml of broth, *without touching the broth*. The broth is not a culture medium. It is used to keep the air around the swab moist so that evaporation and drying of the specimen do not occur. Special culture tubes containing Loeffler's medium are used when diphtheria is suspected. In the latter case, the medium does touch the swab.

In some institutions, culture tubes *without* any fluid are used. These are satisfactory if the specimens are taken to the laboratory without delay.

Laboratory procedure　The swab is to be plated (streaked gently across a dish containing agar). The colonies that grow out will then be identified microscopically or, if necessary, subcultures will be made.

Possible interfering materials and conditions　If the patient has received antibiotics or chemotherapy (such as sulfonamides) there may be a false negative reaction.

Normal range　Many bacteria are normally found in the nose and throat, including pneumococci, staphylococci, streptococci, H. influenzae, K. pneumoniae, and others. The decision as to whether a particular type found in the culture is related to the patient's illness can usually be made only after the physician has correlated these and other findings. The presence of certain types of bacteria, such as those causing tuberculosis or diphtheria, is always abnormal.

Spinal Fluid Culture

The spinal fluid is examined in cases of suspected meningitis. Several kinds of microorganisms may produce meningitis, and precise identification is usually important in order that the most suitable antibiotic may be selected.

Food and drink restrictions　None.

Procedure for collecting specimen　The physician places 2 ml of spinal fluid in a special small test tube. The specimen is stored in an incubator, not a refrigerator.

Laboratory procedure　This is the same as in other cultures. Because of the urgency that exists in the case of meningitis, the laboratory will call the floor as soon as the organism has been identified.

Possible interfering materials and conditions　If the patient has received antibiotics or chemotherapy (such as sulfonamides) there may be a false negative reaction.

Normal range　The spinal fluid is normally sterile.

Sputum Culture

Sputum is material brought up from the lungs and trachea during deep coughing. It should not be confused with saliva or postnasal secretions. This test is often of value in diagnosing lung infections. Since sputum is often contaminated with postnasal secretions and saliva, the organisms found in these secretions may also occur in sputum cultures.

Food and drink restrictions None.

Procedure for collecting specimen The patient uses a special specimen cup or box with a cover. He is instructed to place the sputum raised by a few good coughs into the container. The container is delivered without delay to the bacteriology refrigerator. Containers holding sputum should not be allowed to remain at the bedside for hours. The patient must be warned not to get any sputum on the outside of the container, and it should never be completely filled. If the patient is in isolation, the outside of the container is contaminated and must be handled with the necessary technique to avoid spreading infection.

In some cases, 24-hour sputum specimens are ordered. In such cases, the containers should be replaced well before they are completely filled. Indeed, it may be prudent to leave an extra container with the patient.

Laboratory procedure Essentially the same as with other cultures, with special attention to the presence of acid-fast (tubercle) bacilli.

Possible interfering materials and conditions If the patient has received antibiotics or chemotherapy (such as sulfonamides) there may be a false negative report.

Normal range Both pathogenic and nonpathogenic bacteria are found in some lung diseases. Therefore, after correlating all his findings, the physician must decide whether a particular finding is likely to be significant.

Stool Culture

The normal bacterial flora of the stool is the largest in number and kind found in any part of the body. About 50 varieties of bacteria are normally present in the stool, including several types of pathogenic bacteria. Different culture media are needed for some of the pathogenic bacteria. Therefore, the laboratory should always be told which disease is suspected.

Food and drink restrictions   None.

Procedure for collecting specimen   Use special containers with properly fitted covers. Use a tongue depressor to place a small amount of feces (about 1 inch in diameter) into the container. Avoid contaminating the outside of the container. Deliver promptly to the bacteriology laboratory or refrigerator. Specimens obtained at proctoscopy may be collected on swabs, as described under Nose and Throat Culture.

Laboratory procedure   This will depend on the type of pathogenic bacteria suspected.

Possible interfering materials and conditions   If the patient has received antibiotics or chemotherapy (such as sulfonamides) there may be a false negative reaction.

Normal range   About 50 types of bacteria are normally present in the feces. Some not normally found may be harmless. Usually, specific pathogens such as those of typhoid, dysentery, brucellosis, etc., are sought for and reported if present.

Tests for Special Microorganisms

Certain tests for viral and rickettsial diseases are not ordinarily performed in the hospital laboratory but are sent to a public health department laboratory. In large city health departments or in state public health laboratories tests may be performed for many diseases, including Colorado tick fever, Rocky Mountain spotted fever, influenza, mumps, psittacosis, Q-fever, typhus, and several kinds of virus encephalitis. Tests may also be performed for parasitic infestations such as amebiasis, trichinosis, and echinococcosis. Certain other diseases are tested for by the United States Public Health Laboratory and state laboratories; for example, trypanosomiasis, schistosomiasis, filariasis, leishmaniasis, histoplasmosis, blastomycosis, toxoplasmosis, and leptospirosis.

Procedure for collecting specimen for viral and rickettsial diseases   Two specimens of blood are required. One is drawn during the acute phase of the disease and the other two weeks later. Collect 10 ml of *venous* blood in an appropriate collecting tube. The specimen, needle, and tube are handled with great care to avoid contamination of personnel with infectious agents. Packing the sample for shipment to the appropriate laboratory is done according to the directions of that laboratory. Special containers may usually be obtained from the hospital laboratory.

Treponemal Immobilization Test (TPI)

This is a highly specific test for syphilis with few, if any, false positives, but for technical reasons it is very difficult to perform. It is being replaced by the fluorescent treponemal antibody absorption test.

Urine Culture

Urine culture is often of value in determining the etiological agent in infectious diseases of kidneys, ureters, and bladder.

Food and drink restrictions   None.

Procedure for collecting specimen   In some cases it is possible to collect a sterile noncatheterized specimen from men after cleaning the genital area. However, even with all precautions, some contamination may occur. Therefore, noncatheterized specimens must be brought to the bacteriology laboratory at once, before the contaminating microorganisms multiply and crowd out the pathogens sought. For women patients, it was once customary to use catheterized specimens only. However, recent studies have questioned this procedure. It has been shown that, despite all precautions, the insertion of a catheter into the bladder often introduces infection. *Accordingly, many doctors now believe that it is too risky to catheterize patients for urine culture.* Instead, a clean, voided specimen is used. The entire vulvar area is carefully cleansed, using benzalkonium (Zephiran). It should then be rinsed with sterile water. In place of benzalkonium, a hexachlorophene soap may be used followed by a sterile rinse. However, benzalkonium and hexachlorophene soap should not both be used. The labia are held apart and urine is voided into a sterile bottle. The urine culture is often contaminated by skin bacteria but contamination of the culture is preferable to contamination of the bladder. It is essential to note on the chart whether the urine specimen is passed normally or via catheter.

Laboratory procedure   Essentially the same as in other types of culture.

Possible interfering materials and conditions   If the patient has received antibiotics or chemotherapy (such as sulfonamides) there may be a false negative reaction.

Normal range   Normal urine is sterile. Any bacteria found are contaminants from the skin or invading organisms.

Weil-Felix Test   *See* Agglutination Tests

Widal Test   *See* Agglutination Tests

Wound Culture

When wounds or surgical incisions show evidence of infection, it is frequently important to identify the invading organism so that specific therapy may be instituted.

Food and drink restrictions   None.

Procedure for collecting specimen   The physician collects pus or exudate from the wound on a sterile cotton swab. The swab is placed in a sterile tube as described under Nose and Throat Culture.

Laboratory procedure   The laboratory procedure is generally similar to other cultures. However, special efforts are made to culture anaerobic bacteria, since their presence is serious and requires special handling.

Possible interfering materials and conditions   If the patient has received antibiotics or chemotherapy (such as sulfonamides) there may be a false negative reaction.

Normal range   All wounds and surgical incisions are contaminated by bacteria. However, only a small proportion of them are actually infected. The significance of a culture, therefore, depends on the type of microorganism found and on the clinical picture. Normal skin flora include diphtheroids, E. coli, B. subtilis, P. vulgaris, streptococci, and staphylococci, but others are also found.

3

Tests Performed on Blood

Many tests are performed on blood for diagnostic purposes. When only a drop or two of blood is needed for a test, such as a hemoglobin determination or white blood cell count, it is usually obtained by pricking the finger or ear lobe. This blood oozes from capillaries and is therefore called capillary blood. When a larger quantity is needed, it is obtained from a vein and is called venous blood.

Improper handling of the specimen may give erroneous and misleading results. It is thus essential that in collecting blood for the laboratory the following precautions be observed:

1. The patient should be in the fasting state for several tests. Absorption of food may alter many of the blood constituents. If fats are absorbed, their presence in the blood (lipemia) may interfere with some tests, such as bilirubin, albumin-globulin determination, and others.
2. Hemolysis will cause serious errors in many tests, such as those for potassium, serum bilirubin, and others. Hemolysis is less likely to occur when vacuum containers are used. If a needle and syringe are used, hemolysis can usually be avoided by observing the following precautions:
   a. The syringe must be perfectly dry as well as sterile, since ordinary water will hemolyze red cells.
   b. When drawing the blood, an even pressure should be used in pulling back the plunger of the syringe. Avoid excessive negative pressure.
   c. After drawing the blood, remove the needle from the syringe and empty the latter into the correct container without foaming or splashing the blood.
   d. Do not use containers that have been chilled.
   e. Avoid shaking the specimen unnecessarily.
3. Sometimes, a blood test is ordered on a patient who is receiving an intravenous infusion. A general precaution is

to take blood from the arm *not* receiving the infusion. Nevertheless, this precaution may not always be enough, since it has been reported that when tests were run on blood samples taken when the patient had an intravenous infusion going into the other arm, the results have been distorted. Accordingly, if blood is drawn from a patient while he is receiving an intravenous infusion, that fact should be noted on the patient's chart, and also on the slip sent to the laboratory.

4. Concentration of the blood through venous stasis should be prevented, or some of the tests will give inaccurate results. In order to avoid this, remove the tourniquet from the arm after the needle is definitely in the vein. Allow several seconds to elapse while fresh venous blood fills the vein; then draw the blood into the tube. Unfortunately, this precaution is ignored by many physicians and nurses. As a result, some of the determinations on blood samples drawn by them are inaccurate. The correct procedure is simple and only requires an additional fraction of a minute.

5. After specimens are drawn, send them to the laboratory as soon as possible. If the determinations cannot be made at once, the laboratory is responsible for handling or treating the specimen so that it may be stored safely.

There is increasing use of special disposable vacuum tubes for drawing blood. These have many important advantages over syringes. The vacuum tubes come in various sizes and with different types of anticoagulants for specific tests. They have rubber stoppers of different colors, but unfortunately the manufacturer frequently uses the same color stopper for different kinds of tubes. Therefore, it is important to check the actual serial number of the tube to be sure it is the proper one, rather than to rely completely on the color of the stopper as a guide.

Always draw enough blood into the vacuum tube to fill it. This is particularly important when any test related to blood clotting is to be performed, since inadequate filling of the tube may give spurious results. Unfortunately, some vacuum tubes that remain on the shelf for any length of time may lose part of their vacuum. Such tubes should be discarded at once.

Most tests are designated as "routine." That is, they are performed by the laboratory in the ordinary working schedule. In a few cases it may be necessary to know the results of a particular test as soon as possible. Such specimens are labeled "emergency" or "stat," and the test is carried out at once. The "emergency" or "stat" designation is the responsibility of the physician in charge and should be made only for genuine medical reasons. It is improper to designate a test as an emergency in order to facilitate a patient's early discharge or because the sample was drawn too late for routine testing that day.

When blood or other fluids known or suspected to be harboring a microorganism causing infectious disease are sent, the specimen should be labeled in red, "Infectious Material." Examples are: blood, urine, and stools from typhoid patients; spinal fluid in meningitis; and blood in various rickettsial and viral diseases.

At times, a large number of blood determinations are ordered for a patient on a single day. If the total amount of blood needed for all tests exceeds 20 ml, it may prove difficult or impossible to obtain it from a particular patient, particularly one with poor circulation. Often, the laboratory can manage to perform a satisfactory test with less blood than is usually requested. Therefore, in appropriate cases, it is advisable to call the laboratory in advance and to ask whether they can perform the series of tests with less blood than usual.

A/G (Albumin-Globulin) Ratio *See* Albumin, Globulin, Total Protein, A/G Ratio

Acid Phosphatase *See* Phosphatase, Acid

Albumin, Globulin, Total Protein, A/G Ratio

With the exception of the A/G ratio test, which is now less commonly used than the others, these tests may be useful as aids in the diagnosis of kidney, liver, and some other diseases. They are usually performed on the same blood specimen.

The main function of the serum albumin appears to be the maintenance of osmotic pressure of the blood. The main function of serum globulin is not fully understood, but probably involves immunologic defense. One of its secondary functions is to assist in maintaining the osmotic pressure of the blood. Since the globulin molecule is several times as large as the albumin molecule, it is less efficient, gram for gram, in maintaining osmotic pressure. In certain diseases the albumin may leak out of capillary walls, while the larger globulin molecules are retained within the blood stream. The body may then compensate for loss of albumin by producing more globulin, so that the globulin becomes responsible for a larger share of the osmotic pressure. Yet despite normal or even increased total dissolved protein in the serum, osmotic pressure may be less than normal because of the lesser effectiveness of globulin. As a result, there may be some edema.

Conditions in which the albumin concentration is lowered include chronic nephritis, lipoid nephrosis, liver disease, amyloid nephrosis, and malnutrition.

Food and drink restrictions   None.

Procedure for collecting specimen   Collect 6 ml of *venous* blood in a collecting tube with a red stopper.

Laboratory procedure   The total protein in a sample of serum is determined by the biuret method. Then the albumin is separated from another sample of serum and the amount measured.

Possible interfering materials and conditions   The level of serum proteins may be falsely elevated by Bromsulphalein (BSP). Accordingly, the serum protein measurement should be delayed if the patient has had a BSP test within the past 48 hours.

Normal range   Expressed in gm/100 ml of serum, as listed below.

> *Adults:*   Total serum protein: 6.0 to 8.0
> Serum albumin: 3.2 to 5.6
> Serum globulin: 1.3 to 3.5

> *Children:*   Total serum protein:
> Premature infants: 4.3 to 7.6
> Full-term infants: 4.7 to 7.4
> Other children: 6.0 to 8.0
> Serum albumin: 3.2 to 5.6
> Serum globulin: 2.2 to 3.3

Alcohol

The concentration of blood alcohol in a patient may need to be known for strictly medical or medicolegal purposes. When an unconscious or barely conscious patient is admitted to a hospital, one of the items to be considered in differential diagnosis is alcoholism. In other cases, the level of blood alcohol in a person who is definitely drunk may be helpful in determining the appropriate therapy. With moderate levels, the patient might just be allowed to sleep it off. However, if levels were dangerously high, more vigorous therapy might be indicated.

The medicolegal use of blood alcohol levels is usually based on laws relating to drunken driving. In most areas, highway patrol officers now use devices to measure alcohol concentration in the breath. This indirectly indicates blood levels. However, blood samples may be used in some cases, or a person under arrest may request that his blood be tested as well as his breath.

Blood levels of alcohol under 0.05% mean that the subject is not legally considered to be under the influence of alcohol. However, physiologically, even such low levels reduce driving ability significantly. Levels between 0.05% and 0.15% may or may not be considered to mean that the subject is not legally considered to be under the influence of alcohol. Levels of 0.15% and over are considered clear evidence of being under the influence of alcohol. At levels of 0.25% and over, there is marked intoxication and beginning stupor. At about 0.40%, coma occurs, and at slightly higher levels, death can result.

Food and drink restrictions None.

Procedure for collecting specimen It is essential that no alcohol be used for cleaning the patient's arm. Instead, a *solution* of benzalkonium may be used to clean the venipuncture area, and then wiped off gently with a sterile swab or sponge. A *tincture* must not be used, since it contains alcohol. Collect 5 to 10 ml of *venous* blood in a collecting tube with a green, red, or gray stopper, depending on the particular laboratory. The test is performed on the serum, but it can also be performed on whole blood that has been treated with an anticoagulant.

Laboratory procedure   The sample is subjected to a diffusion or distillation technique to separate the alcohol from the serum or blood. The diffusate or distillate is then added to an acid dichromate solution, producing a color change which can be measured by colorimetry or titration.

Possible interfering materials and conditions   Methyl alcohol (wood alcohol) and isopropyl alcohol can produce measurable levels.

Normal range   Normally there is no alcohol in the blood.

Aldolase, Serum

Aldolase is an enzyme involved in the metabolism of sugars. Its level in the serum is elevated in many disease states, including skeletal muscle disease, cancer, leukemia, megaloblastic anemia, liver diseases, and some other disorders.

Measurement of aldolase level is particularly helpful in diagnosing early cases of Duchenne's muscular dystrophy, in which the level is often substantially elevated even before definite clinical symptoms appear. In the later stages of muscular dystrophy, the levels may return to normal or even go below normal.

Food and drink restrictions   None.

Procedure for collecting specimen   Collect 3 ml of *venous* blood in a collecting tube with a red stopper.

Laboratory procedure   Several methods are available. They are based on the cleavage of a 6-carbon sugar into 3-carbon fractions.

Possible interfering materials and conditions   None reported as yet.

Normal range   *Adults:* This depends on the method used and the hospital. With one method, the normal adult range is 3 to 8 S-L units/100 ml. *Children:* This depends on the method used and the hospital. With one method, the normal children's range is 6 to 16 S-L units/100 ml.

Alkaline Phosphatase   *See* Phosphatase, Alkaline

Ammonia

This is primarily a test of liver function. Ammonia is usually produced by bacterial action in the intestine and is then absorbed into the blood. The liver ordinarily converts the ammonia into urea, which is excreted by the kidneys. When the liver is diseased, its ability to convert ammonia to urea diminishes, and the blood ammonia level rises.

Other conditions that interfere temporarily with liver function may also cause a rise in blood ammonia levels. These include: congestive heart failure, shock, diabetic coma, and severe pneumonia. A change in the vascular pattern such as a portacaval shunt, which permits venous blood from the intestines to bypass the liver and enter the general circulation, could also increase blood ammonia levels.

Food and drink restrictions   None.

Procedure for collecting specimen   Notify the laboratory in advance so that they can be prepared to do the test without delay. Collect 5 ml of *venous* blood in a collecting tube with a green stopper. Fill the tube with blood to its maximum capacity, surround it with ice, and deliver it to the laboratory at once.

Laboratory procedure   Several procedures are in use. One involves diffusing the ammonia into special bottles and adding Nessler's reagent. The result is read by photometer.

Possible interfering materials and conditions   The serum ammonia level may be spuriously elevated by the following drugs:

> acetazolamide (Diamox)
> ammonium salts
> chlorothiazide (Diuril)
> heparin (some brands)
> ion exchange resins (some)
> methicillin (Dimocillin, Staphcillin)
> thiazide drugs
> urea

Normal range   The normal range depends on the techniques used and the experience of the laboratory personnel doing the test, since many factors in the laboratory procedures and timing can influence results. Authoritative sources place the normal range at less than 75 mcg/100 ml of blood. However, in some laboratories the upper limit of normal is considered to be 100 mcg/100 ml of blood.

Amylase

In certain types of pancreatic disease, the digestive enzymes of the pancreas escape into the surrounding tissue, producing necrosis with severe pain and inflammation. Under these circumstances there is an increase in the serum amylase. A serum amylase level of twice normal usually indicates acute pancreatitis. However, there are times when the serum amylase is elevated in abdominal conditions, such as intestinal obstruction. In mumps and other diseases of the salivary glands or ducts, the serum amylase reaches high levels, equivalent to those found in acute pancreatitis.

Some surgeons order routine serum amylase tests for the first few days after any operation that might have injured the pancreas. Whenever an elevation in the amylase level is found, they can institute therapy for pancreatitis early, thus increasing the patient's chances for recovery.

This test remains positive for a short time only, seldom for more than a few days.

Food and drink restrictions   None.

Procedure for collecting specimen   Collect 5 ml of *venous* blood in a collecting tube with a red stopper.

Laboratory procedure   Starch in solution is hydrolyzed by the serum amylase. The amount of reducing sugar present is measured before and after the hydrolysis, and the difference indicates the serum amylase activity.

Possible interfering materials and conditions   Even tiny droplets of saliva contaminating the specimen can cause spurious elevations of amylase readings since saliva has a high concentration of amylase. Therefore, improper pipetting, coughing, sneezing and, when the specimen is in an open container, sometimes even talking near it, either in the patient's room or the laboratory, can result in a misleading reaction.

The amylase levels may be elevated into distinctly abnormal

levels if the patient has received any of the following drugs within 24 hours of drawing the blood sample:

bethanechol (Urecholine)	meperidine (Demerol)
codeine	methyl alcohol [large amounts]
diatrizoate, sodium	methylcholine
ethyl alcohol [large amounts]	morphine
indomethacin (Indocin)	narcotic drugs
	pentazocine (Talwin)

The elevation of serum amylase levels that occurs after the administration of codeine, meperidine (Demerol), or morphine apparently depends on the pancreas being in a state of active secretion when the drugs are given. Therefore, if the patient has not had any food for at least 4 hours before administration of one of these narcotic drugs, an elevated serum amylase level can often be interpreted in the same manner as if a narcotic drug had not been given.

An extremely rare condition, macroamylasemia, may produce elevated serum amylase levels without apparent pancreatitis.

Normal range   80 to 150 units (Somogyi).

Antiglobulin   *See* Coombs' Direct

Antistreptolysin O Titer

This test, usually used in suspected rheumatic fever, indicates the reaction of the body to a recent streptococcal infection. The streptococcus produces many enzymes, one of which, streptolysin O, has the ability to destroy red blood corpuscles. Part of the defense against this bacterium is an antibody that neutralizes streptolysin. Since rheumatic fever is related to a recent streptococcal infection, an increase in the titer of the antistreptolysin is usually found in rheumatic fever. It should be clear, however, that this test, like all others useful in rheumatic fever, is nonspecific and can be positive in many other conditions.

Infants and young children sometimes have normal antistreptolysin titers despite clear-cut rheumatic fever.

Food and drink restrictions   None.

Procedure for collecting specimen   Collect 5 ml of *venous* blood in a collecting tube with a red stopper.

Laboratory procedure   A purified streptolysin from a streptococcus culture is standardized for its ability to dissolve rabbit red blood cells in suspension. Serial dilutions of the patient's serum are then tested to determine the greatest dilution which will prevent this effect of streptolysin.

Possible interfering materials and conditions   None reported yet.

Normal range   Expressed in Todd units /ml of serum, as listed below.

Adults: Up to 160

Children: Newborn: Similar to mother's
6 months to 2 years: Up to 50
2 to 4 years: Up to 160 (probably)
5 to 12 years: Up to 200

APT—Activated Partial Thromboplastin Time   *See* Partial Thromboplastin Time

Antinuclear Antibodies (ANA)

Under certain conditions, the immunological system produces antibodies to the nuclear material in the person's own body. Some of these conditions include systemic lupus erythematosus, progressive systemic sclerosis, rheumatoid arthritis, chronic discoid lupus, dermatomyositis, polyarteritis nodosa, liver cirrhosis, ulcerative colitis, infectious mononucleosis, chronic and acute leukemia, and exposure to certain drugs. Such antibodies may also occur in some normal relatives of patients with systemic lupus erythematosus.

In most of the above-listed conditions, the percentage of patients having antinuclear antibodies is quite varied, but in systemic lupus erythematosus it is close to 100%. Accordingly, this test can sometimes be used to rule out systemic lupus erythematosus. If the test remains negative, the diagnosis of systemic lupus erythematosus is unlikely. On the other hand, a positive test is not of much help, since it occurs in so many situations.

There is some evidence that this test may, in the future, be made more specific. If this occurs, and if a group of similar tests are developed, they are likely to be quite helpful in diagnosing many of these complex diseases.

Food and drink restrictions   None.

Procedure for collecting specimen   Collect 2 ml of *venous* blood in a collecting tube with a red stopper.

Laboratory procedure   The fluorescent antibody technique is used, with microscopic examination under ultraviolet light.

Possible interfering materials and conditions   Hydralazine, isoniazid, procainamide.

Normal range   Normally, there are no antinuclear antibodies in the blood.

Ascorbic Acid (Vitamin C)

This test is being performed much less often now than in the past, but it remains an important diagnostic tool. Ascorbic acid is an essential vitamin found in fresh fruits and vegetables. Deficiencies are not uncommon, and may even occur in persons who are on an apparently adequate diet and are taking vitamin supplements. The severe deficiency, scurvy, is rare and is usually readily recognized. However, relative deficiencies may occur in several conditions and interfere with recovery. For example, in patients with severe burns, the need for ascorbic acid is markedly increased. The same may be true of those with severe infections. In some cancer patients, through mechanisms that are not clear, the ascorbic acid level may be quite low despite an adequate diet and presumably therapeutic supplements of the vitamin. This fact may be important, since ascorbic acid is vital to the body's defense mechanisms. For all these reasons, it is often helpful to know the patient's ascorbic acid level.

Food and drink restrictions   None.

Procedure for collecting specimen   Collect 5 ml of *venous* blood in a collecting tube with a gray stopper.

Laboratory procedure   Several different methods are available. Most of them are based on the ability of ascorbic acid to decolorize a solution made blue by the addition of a special reagent.

Possible interfering materials and conditions   None reported yet.

Normal range 0.6 to 1.6 mg/100 ml of blood plasma.

Ascorbic Acid (Vitamin C) Tolerance (Blood) *See also* Ascorbic Acid Tolerance (Urine)

This test measures the degree of ascorbic acid deficiency. Although it is not as widely performed as in the past, it can provide important clinical information since some persons with seemingly adequate diets, and even some receiving supplemental vitamins, may have a partial deficiency of ascorbic acid. This may be true of patients with severe burns, infection, or malignancy. A partial deficiency of ascorbic acid can interfere with wound healing, body defenses, and recovery.

Food and drink restrictions For 24 hours before the test, the patient must avoid foods high in ascorbic acid. Water may be taken as desired.

Procedure for collecting specimen The physician administers 10 mg/kg of ascorbic acid as a 4% solution in sterile saline intravenously. Four hours after the injection, 5 ml of *venous* blood are collected in a collecting tube with a gray stopper.

The test is performed on plasma and may be done in conjunction with the urine test (p. 136).

Laboratory procedure The amount of ascorbic acid is measured photometrically after chemical modification.

Possible interfering materials and conditions High potency vitamin supplements.

Normal range 1.6 mg/100 ml or higher.

ASO Titer *See* Antistreptolysin O Titer (Blood)

Australia Antigen Assay

This is a test performed by blood banks to determine whether donor blood contains the virus of serum hepatitis. The relationship between Australia antigen and the hepatitis virus is not yet proven, but they are likely to be identical. Most blood banks now test all donor blood for Australia antigen and discard those blood units that are positive.

Since serum hepatitis is the most serious complication of blood transfusions, with a mortality rate of 5 to 10%, it is vital to be able to detect blood that can cause this disease. In volunteer blood donors, between 1 and 2 in every 1,000 are positive; in commercial blood donors, 10 to 12 in every 1,000 are positive. Since millions of blood transfusions are given each year, the saving in lives and disability from eliminating the contaminated blood from banks is substantial. Every blood bank should employ this test routinely on each and every unit of blood. False positives are virtually unknown, and false negatives are rare. The test is generally performed on bank blood that has already been drawn from the donor.

Food and drink restrictions None.

Procedure for collecting specimen This is done by the blood bank.

Laboratory procedure A common procedure is radioimmunoassay.

Possible interfering materials and conditions Interfering materials are not yet reported. Interfering conditions that may produce false positives in the donor blood include leukemia, Down's syndrome (mongolism), leprosy, and chronic renal disease, but patients with these conditions ought not be blood donors anyway.

Normal range *Adults:* Negative. *Children:* Children are not used as blood donors, so this test is not usually performed on their blood.

Bacillus Subtilis Inhibition *See* Guthrie

Barbiturate

Barbiturate levels in the serum of unconscious patients are measured when there is a possibility of accidental or suicidal ingestion of an overdose of barbiturate. If high levels are found, therapy can be directed in a more meaningful way at the cause of the unconsciousness. The evaluation of the significance of high barbiturate levels is complicated by several factors. Other drugs, including tranquilizers and alcohol, can intensify the effects of moderate levels of barbiturates. Furthermore, the available tests do not yet permit the doctor to tell exactly which barbiturate has been ingested, and different barbiturates produce coma at different blood levels. The long-acting barbiturates such as phenobarbital (Luminal) produce coma at blood levels of about 8 mg/100 ml. The medium-duration barbiturates such as amobarbital (Amytal) require levels of about 4 mg/100 ml, and the short-acting barbiturates such as secobarbital (Seconal) and pentobarbital (Nembutal) require levels of only about 2 to 2.5 mg/100 ml to produce coma. Measurement of blood barbiturate level is almost always done on an emergency basis.

Food and drink restrictions   None.

Procedure for collecting specimen   Collect 5 to 10 ml of *venous* blood in a collecting tube with a green or red stopper, depending on the laboratory.

Laboratory procedure   The serum is extracted with chloroform, and alkali is added to the extract. Differential ultraviolet spectrophotometry is then used to measure barbiturate concentration.

Possible interfering materials and conditions   The barbiturate level may be spuriously elevated by antipyrine and by theophylline in large doses.

Normal range   Normally, there are no barbiturates in the blood.

Bilirubin, Partition (Direct and Indirect van den Bergh Test)

This test is becoming less common. When the ability of the liver to excrete bilirubin is impaired by obstruction, either within or outside the organ, it is believed that the excess circulating bilirubin is free of any attached protein. However, when the increase in circulating bilirubin is due to increased destruction of red blood cells (hemolysis), it is believed that the bilirubin is bound to protein. By measuring the amount of free bilirubin (direct) and the amount bound to protein (indirect), there is some indication as to whether the patient's illness is based on obstruction or hemolysis.

Food and drink restrictions   None.

Procedure for collecting specimen   Collect 5 ml of *venous* blood in a collecting tube with a red stopper.

Laboratory procedure   The direct method is described below. In the indirect method, alcohol is added to the sample of serum. The serum proteins precipitate, freeing any bilirubin that was bound to them, and the bilirubin dissolves in the alcohol. Ehrlich's reagent is then added to the alcoholic extract and the intensity of the color produced is measured.

Possible interfering materials and conditions   The serum bilirubin may be spuriously high if the patient has had foods or drugs that impart an orange or yellow color to the serum. There may also be elevated levels when the patient has taken drugs that temporarily modify liver function. In such cases, the elevated levels may be real rather than spurious, but they do not indicate liver disease. The materials in both categories are listed below, by official (generic) name only, because of the large number involved:

acetohexamide
anabolic agents, some
androgens, some
aspidium
carotene
carrots
chlordiazepoxide
erythromycin
indomethacin
isoniazid
lipochrome
menadiol (large amounts)
mercaptopurine
methanol
nitrofurantoin
novobiocin

oxacillin
phenothiazines
phytonadione
pipobroman
pyrazinamide
quinacrine
radiopaque contrast media, some
salicylates (large amounts)
sulfonamides
triacetyloleandomycin
trifluperidol
vitamin A
vitamin K in large doses in newborn

Normal range   *Adults:* 0.1 to 1.0 mg/100 ml. Within the normal range, the ratio between the amounts of bilirubin found on direct and indirect measurements is of no significance. When the concentration of bilirubin rises significantly over 1.0 mg/100 ml, the relative amounts that are free and bound to protein may suggest the type of disorder. If most of the bilirubin is found on the direct test, the chances are that the patient has an obstructive lesion. If most of it is found on the indirect test, the illness is likely to be hemolytic in origin. These interpretations indicate probabilities, not certainties, and there is some controversy about the meaning of these tests. *Children:* 0.2 to 0.8 mg/100 ml.

Bilirubin, Total

Bilirubin is derived from the hemoglobin in red blood cells that have been broken down. Constantly being produced, it is excreted by the liver into the bile, of which it is the chief pigment. There is always a small amount in the serum. When the destruction of red blood cells becomes excessive or when the liver is unable to excrete the ordinary quantities of bilirubin produced, the concentration in the serum rises. If the concentration becomes very high, there is visible jaundice. It is advantageous to discover the increased concentration of serum bilirubin before jaundice is seen, and that is accomplished by this test.

Food and drink restrictions   None.

Procedure for collecting specimen   Collect 5 ml of *venous* blood in a collecting tube with a red stopper.

Laboratory procedure   Ehrlich's reagent is added to the sample of serum. A colored product is formed and the intensity of the color is used as a measure of the bilirubin concentration.

Possible interfering materials and conditions   The serum bilirubin may be spuriously high if the patient has had foods or drugs that impart an orange or yellow color to the serum. There may also be elevated levels when the patient has taken drugs that temporarily modify liver function. In such cases, the elevated levels may be real rather than spurious, but they do not indicate liver disease. The materials in both categories are listed below, by official (generic) name only, because of the large number involved:

acetohexamide
anabolic agents, some
androgens, some
aspidium
carotene
carrots
chlordiazepoxide
erythromycin
indomethacin
isoniazid
lipochrome
menadiol (large amounts)

mercaptopurine
methanol
nitrofurantoin
novobiocin
oxacillin
phenothiazines
phytonadione
pipobroman
pyrazinamide
quinacrine
radiopaque contrast
   media, some

salicylates (large
    amounts)
sulfonamides
triacetyloleandomycin

trifluperidol
vitamin A
vitamin K in large doses
    in newborn

Normal range *Adults:* 0.1 to 1.0 mg/100 ml of serum. *Children:* 0.2 to 0.8 mg/100 ml of serum.

Bleeding Time

This test measures the time during which there is bleeding from a small skin incision. It is quite distinct from tests for clotting time and gives somewhat different information since, in a bleeding time test, constriction of the small vessels is also involved. Bleeding time is prolonged in thrombocytopenic purpura and other blood disorders.

Food and drink restrictions None.

Procedure for performing test and collecting specimen A standardized puncture wound of the skin is produced with an appropriate instrument. The site of the puncture may be the finger tip, ear lobe, or forearm. In some variations when the arm is used, a blood pressure cuff increases the venous pressure to make the test more sensitive. After the puncture is produced, the drops of blood are wiped away with filter paper every 30 seconds. The time at which bleeding stops is recorded.

Possible interfering materials and conditions None reported yet.

Normal range 1 to 6 minutes.

Blood Counts

Frequently, various blood cell and platelet counts are ordered either routinely to help with a particular problem or to follow the results of treatment. Several counts are often performed together and will, therefore, be considered together here. Blood counts are performed on whole blood, usually capillary blood, although venous blood can be used.

Although the procedures described here are basic and still in wide use, they are rapidly being supplanted by electronic counters in most large institutions.

Complete blood count (CBC) refers to red cell count, white cell count, and white cell differential count.

Platelet Count

The platelets (thrombocytes), which are necessary for the clotting of blood, are particles much smaller than red blood cells. They are reduced in such conditions as thrombocytopenic purpura, aplastic anemia, Gaucher's disease, and septicemia. They may be increased in polycythemia, fractures, and certain kinds of anemia.

Food and drink restrictions   None.

Procedure for performing test and collecting specimen   The procedure is essentially the same as for red blood cell counts, but employs a special diluting fluid.

Possible interfering materials and conditions   None reported yet.

Normal range   *Adult:* 150,000 to 400,000 per cu mm. *Children:* At birth, and during first week, level is close to 150,000 per cu mm. It then rises rapidly into the adult range.

Red Cell Count

The red cells (erythrocytes) contain hemoglobin, the essential oxygen carrier of the blood. An increase in red cells may indicate hemoconcentration (insufficient water in the blood), or polycythemia, a condition characterized by a persistently elevated red cell count. A reduction in the red cell count may come from hemorrhage or one of the anemias.

Food and drink restrictions   None.

Procedure for performing test and collecting specimen   In the older method, the finger or ear lobe is punctured and blood is drawn into a special red cell pipette, up to a given mark. Diluting solution is then added up to a second mark, and the contents thoroughly mixed. The diluted suspension is then allowed to flow into a space in a special counting chamber. Through the use of a microscope, the cells per unit area are then counted and the number of cells calculated. Newer methods use electronic counters.

Possible interfering materials and conditions None reported yet.

Normal range Expressed in numbers of red cells per cubic millimeter (cu mm). Note that this unit of volume is only 1/1000 of a ml or a cc.

Adults: 4,000,000 to 6,000,000

Children: Newborn: The count depends to some extent on when the umbilical cord was clamped. If the cord was clamped late in delivery, red cell counts are significantly higher than if the cord was clamped early. Capillary counts tend to be higher than counts of venous blood.
1 day to 2 weeks: 3,500,000 to 8,200,000
2 weeks to 3 months: Gradual fall to lower level of adult range
3 months to 2 years: Gradual rise to adult levels

Reticulocyte Count

This test gives some indication of bone marrow activity. Reticulocytes are immature red blood cells. They retain a network of reticular material that can be stained with the proper dyes. When the bone marrow cells are very active (a situation that occurs after hemorrhage and with recovery from anemia), there is an increase in the number of reticulocytes in the blood. When the bone marrow cells are less active, the number of reticulocytes in the blood falls.

This test is often performed to evaluate the response to anemia therapy.

Food and drink restrictions None.

Procedure for performing test and collecting specimen A thin film of cresyl blue is allowed to dry on a glass slide. A fresh drop of blood is then spread over the stain and kept moist to allow the stain to penetrate the cells. Using a microscope, the number of reticulocytes per 1,000 red blood cells is determined.

Possible interfering materials and conditions None reported yet.

Normal range *Adults:* 0.1 to 1.5 reticulocytes per 100 red blood cells. *Children:* Probably similar to the range for adults, but this has not been definitely established.

White Cell Count

White blood cells (leucocytes) are important in the defense of the body against invading microorganisms, since they destroy most harmful bacteria. An increase in the count is usually seen in infections. It may also be observed in other conditions, including emotional upsets, blood disorders, and anesthesia. A decrease in the white blood cells may be seen in blood dyscrasias, overwhelming infections, and drug and chemical toxicity.

Food and drink restrictions None.

Procedure for performing test and collecting specimen Essentially the same as for the red blood cell count, but a different pipette is used with a special diluting solution to hemolyze the red cells. Newer methods use electronic counters.

Possible interfering materials and conditions None reported yet.

Normal range Expressed in numbers of white cells per cubic millimeter (cu mm), as listed below.

Adults: 4,000 to 11,000

Children: Newborn: 9,000 to 35,000
2 months to 2 years: 6,000 to 18,000
After 2 years: Gradual fall to adult levels

White Cell Differential Count

Several kinds of white blood cells (leucocytes) can be identified microscopically. It is often helpful to know whether the proportions of these cells in the blood have changed, inasmuch as that may direct attention to a particular group of diseases. The neutrophiles (neutral-staining multinucleated cells) are increased in most bacterial infections. The eosinophiles (acid-staining multinucleated cells) are increased in parasitic infestations and allergic conditions. The basophiles (basic-staining multinucleated cells) may be increased in some blood dyscrasias. The lymphocytes may be increased in measles and in several bacterial infections. The monocytes may be increased during recovery from severe infections, Hodgkin's disease, and lipoid storage diseases. The reasons for these changes are not known.

Food and drink restrictions   None.

Procedure for performing test and collecting specimen   A drop of fresh blood is placed on a slide and a second slide is used to spread the blood evenly over the surface of the glass in a thin film. After the film has dried, it is stained and examined under the microscope. Each type of white blood cell is counted separately. A total of 100 white cells of all kinds is counted, and the relative percentage of each calculated.

Possible interfering materials and conditions   None reported yet.

Normal range

Adults:	Neutrophiles	54% to 62%
	Eosinophiles (acidophiles)	1% to 3%
	Basophiles	0% to 1%
	Lymphocytes	25% to 33%
	Monocytes	0% to 9%

Children: Newborns tend to have differentials that approach adult patterns. By the fourth day of life, neutrophiles have usually dropped to about 40 to 50% and lymphocytes have risen to about 45%. From then on, there is a gradual shift to the adult ratio, which is reached at about age 19 to 21.

Blood Gases   *See* Carbon Dioxide, PCO_2, and PO_2

Blood Types

Blood typing tests are important in patients who may need blood transfusions and in pregnant women. There are four main blood types, A, B, AB, and O, and several minor types. The letters refer to the kind of agglutinogen present in the red blood cells. Type A blood has A agglutinogen, B has B agglutinogen. AB has both A and B agglutinogen, and O has no agglutinogen. Each person has in his *serum* the agglutinins that react with all types of agglutinogen *not* present in his own cells. Thus, A blood has anti-B agglutinin, B blood has anti-A agglutinin, AB has *no* agglutinin, and O has both anti-A and anti-B agglutinins. Whenever agglutinins in sufficient concentration come in contact with the corresponding agglutinogen, agglutination (clumping) of the red cells occurs, followed by rapid destruction of these cells. This often causes death. Thus, if A blood is mixed with B or O type in equal amounts, the anti-A agglutinins in the other blood will clump and destroy the A cells. In most cases of incompatible transfusion, the *donor's* cells are agglutinated by the recipient's (patient's) serum, rather than the reverse. The reason for this is that in a transfusion 500 ml of donor's blood are added to approximately 5000 ml of recipient's blood. The donor's blood is, therefore, diluted approximately 10 times. This weakens the agglutinins of the donor's blood so that ordinarily they cannot agglutinate red cells. However, the agglutinins of the recipient's blood are only diluted by 10%, and remain strong. The dilution of the donor's blood does not affect the agglutinogens of the donor's red cells. Thus, the agglutinins of the recipient will clump the red cells of the donor in most incompatible transfusions. Exceptions occur only in those cases in which the donor has an unusually high concentration of agglutinins in his serum (higher titer). In these rare cases the donor's agglutinins are powerful enough to remain active even after a 1:10 dilution and will clump the recipient's red cells.

Persons with type O blood are usually referred to as "universal donors." This is a misnomer, resulting from past practices. In the past, type O blood was sometimes given in emergencies. (Rarely, it might be justifiable to give it still in unusual emergencies, but these do not occur in usual hospital settings.) If more than one unit of O blood is transfused, the risk of a transfusion reaction goes up steeply with each additional unit, since the dilution of donor serum becomes less and less.

For a similar reason, persons with AB blood are called "universal recipients." Here too, if the titer of the agglutinins in the donor's blood is high, a severe or even fatal reaction may occur. The same considerations and precautions that apply to the use of "universal donor" blood also apply, therefore, to the use of blood of different types for "universal recipients."

In recent years additional blood types have been found and probably more will be discovered. These other types exist in conjunction with the main groups and the Rh groups. Their importance is much less, although they have theoretical interest and are sometimes used with the other groups in cases of disputed paternity.

Rh Factor

The Rh factor is found in conjunction with any one of the main blood types. A person may be ARh+, ARh−, BRh+, BRh−, etc. The presence of the Rh factor is designated Rh+, its absence Rh−. The same considerations that apply to the main groups also apply to the Rh groups in transfusions. The Rh groups differ from the main blood groups in two important respects. First, the serum of an Rh− person does not ordinarily have significant amounts of anti-Rh agglutinins, unless there has been previous exposure to Rh+ blood. The previous exposure may have been a transfusion or injection of Rh+ blood, or pregnancy with an Rh+ fetus. With exposure to Rh+ blood, the Rh− person gradually builds up a high titer of anti-Rh agglutinins. The second difference between the Rh and main blood groupings is that in some cases anti-Rh agglutinin readily crosses the placental barrier, while the main agglutinins apparently do not usually do so in significant quantities. The importance of these aspects of the Rh factor lies not only in the area of blood transfusions but also in pregnancy. The occurrence of erythroblastosis fetalis (destruction of the infant's red cells) in Rh+ babies born to Rh− mothers is commonly known and greatly exaggerated. Because of the need for prior exposure to Rh+ blood before large amounts of anti-Rh agglutinins are produced, the first Rh+ child of an Rh− mother will almost always be normal unless the mother has had a transfusion or injection of Rh+ blood. Also, many Rh− women have several normal Rh+ children, since there is considerable variation in the titer of anti-Rh agglutinin produced by different individuals and also in the amounts of anti-Rh agglutinin which pass the placental barrier.

Over 90% of all infants born with erythroblastosis come from Rh negative mothers who have produced anti-Rh antibodies. The remainder result from immunization of the mother to one of the major blood groups (A and B) or to one of the minor blood groups.

In some hospitals, women with Rh− blood are tested for rising titer of anti-Rh antibodies. This is sometimes, but not always, helpful in predicting the occurrence of erythroblastosis in the infant.

The Rh antigen is now referred to as the D antigen by some authorities.

Food and drink restrictions   None.

Procedure for collecting specimen   Collect 5 ml of *venous* blood in a collecting tube with a red stopper.

Laboratory procedure   There are several methods of typing blood, each with its own advantages and disadvantages. In general, all methods depend on the mixing of the patient's red cells with separate standard serum samples of groups A and B. As an additional check, the patient's serum is mixed with red cell suspensions of A and also of B types. The type of serum that agglutinates the patient's red cells and the type of red cell agglutinated by the patient's serum indicate the patient's blood type. A similar test is used to distinguish between Rh− and Rh+ blood. False positive as well as false negative reactions can occur, so that these tests are entrusted to a skilled and experienced person. A mistake in blood typing may be responsible for the death of the patient.

Possible interfering materials and conditions   None reported yet.

Bromides

This test is performed to determine whether certain symptoms, including coma, could be due to excess bromide ingestion. The use of bromides by physicians for sedation has declined almost to the vanishing point. However, some over-the-counter medicines still contain bromides and toxicity from cumulative overdosage still occurs.

Food and drink restrictions   None reported.

Procedure for collecting specimen   Collect 5 ml of *venous* blood in a collecting tube with a green stopper.

Laboratory procedure   A colorimetric test is used.

Possible interfering materials and conditions   None reported yet.

Normal range   *Adults:* Normally, there is no measurable bromide in the serum. Low levels indicate ingestion but not necessarily toxicity. Levels over 100 mg/100 ml of serum are usually found when there are toxic symptoms. *Children:* Same as for adults.

Blood Urea Nitrogen (BUN)   *See* Urea Nitrogen

Bromsulphalein Retention (BSP)

This is a sensitive test for liver function. When Bromsulphalein is injected intravenously, about 80% of it is removed by the liver and about 20% by other organs. If the liver does not function properly, more than the normal amount of the injected Bromsulphalein will remain in the blood. If marked jaundice is present, the test cannot be performed satisfactorily and is not needed.

Recently, evidence has been obtained that Bromsulphalein is an irritant to the veins, and that in about 15% of cases, some venous induration will occur, apparently on the basis of local thrombophlebitis. Accordingly, there have been warnings against use of the test except for clearly defined reasons.

Bromsulphalein may be particularly hazardous in patients with asthma.

There have also been reports of serious and fatal sensitivity reactions to Bromsulphalein. *Therefore, it is recommended that on the injection tray there be an extra syringe and needle, and an ampul of epinephrine.*

Food and drink restrictions   The patient must fast for 12 hours before the test. Water is permitted.

Procedure for collecting specimen   The patient cannot receive any other dyes for 2 days before the test, and must fast for 12 hours.

The solution must *not* be refrigerated and should be at room temperature. The vial should be examined in good light for possible crystals before the contents are injected. The injection itself should be done slowly, taking a full 3 minutes. The patient is weighed just before the test and 5 mg of Bromsulphalein dye per kg of body weight is injected intravenously by the physician. It is essential that none of the dye be allowed to leak into the tissues, since it is highly irritating and causes sloughing. After exactly 45 minutes have passed, 7 ml of *venous* blood is drawn from the opposite arm into a collecting tube with a red stopper.

Laboratory procedure   The amount of Bromsulphalein in the serum sample is determined colorimetrically. Marked jaundice will make the measurements unsatisfactory.

Possible interfering materials and conditions   The BSP may be artificially elevated if the patient has taken any of a large variety of drugs. Because of the number of drugs involved, they are listed mainly by official (generic) name, with only a few prominent brand names included:

Amidone
anabolic steroids
  (see Table 16)
androgens (See Table 16)
antifungal agents
aspidium
azo drugs (see Table 17)
barbiturates (see Table 18)
Bunamiodyl
chlorpropamide
chlortetracycline
choleretics
clofibrate
clomiphene
contraceptives, oral
dyes for gallbladder studies
estradiol
estriol
estrogens (see Table 21)
Ethoxazene
florantyrone

fluoxymesterone
heparin
iopanoic acid
isocarboxazid
MAO inhibitors
meperidine (Demerol)
metaxalone
methandrostenolone
methotrexate
methyldopa
methyltestosterone
morphine
norethandrolone
norethindrone
oxacillin
Pethidine
phenazopyridine
phenolphthalein
probenecid
tolbutamide
triacetyloleandomycin

Normal range   *Adults:* Less than 0.4 mg of Bromsulphalein per 100 ml of serum. If expressed as % retention, the normal level is less than 5%. *Children:* This test is not commonly performed on children.

BSP   *See* Bromsulphalein Retention

BT   *See* Bleeding Time

BUN   *See* Urea Nitrogen

Calcium

Calcium is one of the essential ions in the body. It is needed for many vital processes such as muscular contraction, nerve transmission, and blood clotting. The minimum concentration of calcium ions required for each of these processes differs somewhat. Only ionized calcium is effective, and measurement of ionized calcium levels is still a research procedure. However, the total amount of calcium, ionized and nonionized, can be determined. It is generally believed that about 50% of the total calcium is ionized. If there is any acidosis, the percentage of ionized calcium is higher. In alkalosis, the percentage of ionized calcium is lower. The total calcium level alone does not indicate the amount of ionized calcium.

When there is a deficiency in ionized calcium, the major manifestation is a generalized tetanic condition beginning with twitching of muscle fibers and finally producing tetanic convulsions. This condition is probably due to the response of the nerves or neuromuscular junctions to the reduced calcium levels. It is unlikely that blood clotting changes are related to calcium levels, since normal clotting can take place at calcium levels considerably lower than those that would be fatal because of the production of severe, sustained tetanic convulsions. Therefore, calcium determinations are of no value in disorders of blood clotting.

A decrease in the blood calcium, called hypocalcemia, occurs in several conditions. In celiac disease and sprue, absorption of calcium from the gastrointestinal tract is impaired. In hypoparathyroidism, the balance between blood calcium and bone calcium is disturbed, and in some kidney diseases excess calcium is lost in the urine.

An increase in the blood calcium (hypercalcemia) is found in a number of conditions, including hyperparathyroidism (overfunctioning of the parathyroids), multiple myeloma, and respiratory diseases with increased carbon dioxide tension (concentration) in the blood.

Food and drink restrictions   None.

Procedure for collecting specimen   Collect 5 ml of *venous* blood in a collecting tube with a red stopper.

Laboratory procedure   Several methods are available. The preferred method is atomic absorption spectrophotometry when the needed instruments are available.

Possible interfering materials and conditions   The serum calcium level may be spuriously decreased if the patient has had a BSP retention test during the previous 24 to 48 hours.

A number of drugs may interfere with the calcium measurement, making it difficult or impossible to obtain a correct reading. They include heparin, insulin, and magnesium salts.

Normal range   Expressed in milligrams per 100 milliliters (mg/100 ml) or milliequivalents per liter (mEq/L).

Adults: 9.0 to 11.4 mg/100 ml *or*
4.5 to 5.7 mEq/L

Children: Newborn to 1 week: 7.4 to 14.0 mg/100 ml *or*
3.7 to 7.0 mEq/L

Over 1 week: 9.0 to 12.0 mg/100 ml *or*
4.5 to 6.0 mEq/L

Carbon Dioxide (CO_2)

Carbon dioxide levels in plasma are measured in cases of suspected respiratory insufficiency. A higher than normal concentration of carbon dioxide may indicate that gas exchange is inadequate. This test is often performed and interpreted in conjunction with the oxygen level (p. 98) and pH (p. 94) of the plasma.

Carbon dioxide levels are ordinarily measured in *venous* plasma. Under some circumstances, arterial carbon dioxide levels may be measured. The arterial levels are normally slightly different from venous levels, and the technique of obtaining arterial blood is more difficult, usually requiring a specially trained physician.

The physician may designate carbon dioxide level measurement "emergency."

Food and drink restrictions   None.

Procedure for collecting specimen   There are several procedures in general use, and the laboratory should be consulted to determine the type of container to collect the blood in. In all procedures, the patient must avoid clenching his fist or exercising his arm, since this can raise the carbon dioxide level in the blood.

Some laboratories want the blood collected in a heparinized vacutainer tube; others prefer a heparinized syringe that is immediately put on ice; still others require a sample collected in a vacutainer tube without anticoagulant. In all cases, the container must be completely filled with blood. No air can be permitted to get into the container. The color of the stopper of the collecting tube varies from laboratory to laboratory.

Laboratory procedure   The sample is acidified, and the carbon dioxide gas extracted and measured in a gasometer.

Possible interfering materials and conditions   The test for carbon dioxide content may be interfered with if the patient has received dimercaprol, lipomul, or methicillin.

There may be a spurious decrease in carbon dioxide content if the patient has received nitrofurantoin.

Inadvertent exposure of the sample to outside air may give erroneous results. Exercise of the hand and forearm muscles may produce spurious elevations.

Normal range   The normal range for *venous* plasma carbon dioxide as given by several authorities varies somewhat. Some give fairly narrow limits, others wider ones. The following range encompasses most of the figures given:

$$22 \text{ to } 34 \text{ mM/L } or$$
$$22 \text{ to } 34 \text{ mEq/L } or$$
$$50 \text{ to } 60 \text{ vol } \%$$

The normal range for *arterial* plasma carbon dioxide is 21 to 30 mM/ *or* mEq/L.

Carbon Dioxide Combining Power   *See* CO_2 Combining Power

Carbon Monoxide (CO)

Carbon monoxide has a much greater affinity for hemoglobin than either oxygen or carbon dioxide. Hemoglobin that comes in contact with carbon monoxide forms carboxyhemoglobin, which cannot transport oxygen or carbon dioxide. This accounts for the toxicity of carbon monoxide.

In suspected carbon monoxide poisoning, the identification of increased amounts of carboxyhemoglobin in the blood establishes the diagnosis. The test is not restricted to acute carbon monoxide poisoning, which frequently has a fatal outcome before the doctor arrives. There are many cases of chronic, low grade carbon monoxide poisoning causing such symptoms as headache, malaise, and weakness. They are not easily diagnosed except by determination of the blood carbon monoxide level. Poisoning usually results from occupational exposure to exhaust gases in industrial plants, garages, etc. It may also come from defective gas-burning appliances in the home. Most persons have small amounts of carbon monoxide in their blood from exposure to tobacco smoke, automobile exhaust fumes, etc.

There have been tragic deaths because this test was omitted on persons who came to hospital clinics in the winter complaining of headache. In at least one case, the patient went home, and the defective gas heater whose carbon monoxide output caused the headache killed all but one of the family that night.

Food and drink restrictions None.

Procedure for collecting specimen Collect *venous* blood in a collecting tube with a lavender stopper. Seven (7) ml are needed usually, but there are micromethods available that require much less blood. The laboratory should be consulted.

Laboratory procedure Several laboratory procedures are available. A usual method is quantitative estimation using a spectroscope.

Possible interfering materials and conditions None reported yet.

Normal range Technically, there should only be traces of carbon monoxide in the blood. However, almost all people are exposed to some carbon monoxide from automobile exhausts, smokers, and so forth. Studies have shown that levels of up to 1 g of carboxyhemoglobin per 100 ml of blood are not uncommon in city dwellers and do not represent a known hazard.

CBC   *See* Blood Counts

Carcinoembryonic Antigen Assay (CEA)

This test is used to follow the results of treatment in patients with cancer. Its exact significance is not yet known. The test is *not* useful in diagnosing cancer, since elevated titers are found in many conditions other than cancer. The antigen is found in embryos and in extracts of some cancers. It is also found in several noncancerous disorders of the gastrointestinal tract. When a patient is known to have cancer, a baseline assay of the carcinoembryonic antigen level is taken. Then, following treatment, additional measurements are made at about 30- to 60-day intervals. When levels fall below 2.5 ng/ml and remain there, the tumor is probably under control, although not necessarily eradicated. A significant rise in levels after an interval suggests a recurrence before clinical symptoms appear, thus permitting the physician to start or resume chemotherapy sooner. For 30 days following surgery, there is commonly a moderate rise in titer that is considered to have no prognostic significance. The test is still rather new and it is not known definitely which kinds of cancer it is useful for. At this time, it seems to be definitely helpful in following cancers of colon, rectum, and pancreas. It may also prove helpful in following others.

Food and drink restrictions   None.

Procedure for collecting specimen   Collect *venous* blood in a collecting tube with a lavender stopper. The tube should be filled to rated capacity, so that the vacuum is eliminated.

Laboratory procedure   A radioimmunoassay procedure is used.

Possible interfering materials and conditions   Heparin may interfere with the test. Accordingly, the test should not be done on patients who have received heparin during the preceding 2 days, and under no circumstances should heparin be allowed to come in contact with the blood sample.

Normal range   *Adults:* The exact limits of the normal range are not known. In general, levels below 2.5 ng/ml (nanograms/milliliter) are not considered significant. *Children:* This test is not ordinarily performed on children. It is possible that some newborn infants might still have traces of carcinoembryonic antigen from fetal life, but it should be at a low level by the age of a few months.

Carotene

This is primarily a screening test for disorders of intestinal absorption. Carotene is a normal component of green and yellow vegetables, particularly carrots. It is a precursor of vitamin A. In disorders of intestinal absorption, carotene levels are depressed.

Food and drink restrictions Restrictions will depend on the doctor's orders. If he wishes to know the carotene level without added dietary carotene, green and yellow vegetables and vegetable juices should be omitted for 3 days before the test. On the other hand, sometimes the doctor may wish to check levels after the patient has been on a diet high in carotene and will order a diet containing carotene.

Procedure for collecting specimen Collect *venous* blood in a collecting tube with a red stopper. Different hospital laboratories require different amounts, ranging from 4 to 10 ml.

Laboratory procedure This varies from laboratory to laboratory.

Possible interfering materials and conditions Mineral oil interferes with carotene absorption.

Normal range *Adults:* This varies from hospital to hospital. In general, levels of 40 to 300 micrograms/100 ml are considered normal. Levels under 30 micrograms/100 ml usually indicate serious depletion or inadequate absorption. *Children:* The diet of young infants may be low in carotene, and this test is not usually done on them. Normal levels for infants and children are not established.

CEA   *See* Carcinoembryonic Antigen Assay

Cephalin Flocculation

This test was once commonly used in diagnosing liver damage. However, in many hospitals it is now being replaced with more specific enzyme studies of liver functions.

The serum of normal persons, properly diluted, will not flocculate (clump) a colloidal suspension of cephalin and cholesterol. On the other hand, the serum of persons whose liver cells are damaged does flocculate the suspension. This test is sensitive and is frequently positive in the early stages of liver disease before jaundice appears. It is negative in acute biliary tract obstruction of short duration. If the obstruction persists, secondary damage to the liver cells occurs and the cephalin flocculation test becomes positive. Certain types of liver disease that do not damage the liver cells give a negative reaction, for example, neoplasms and abscesses. Some nonhepatic disorders, such as malaria, kala-azar, and rheumatoid arthritis, may sometimes produce a positive reaction. A positive test, therefore, is not itself conclusive. Since this test affords a rough quantitative measurement of liver cell function, it is sometimes used to follow the course of patients with a known liver disease, such as cirrhosis. The results are reported as negative to 4+.

Food and drink restrictions None.

Procedure for collecting specimen Collect 5 ml of *venous* blood in a collecting tube with a red stopper.

Laboratory procedure A 1:20 dilution of the serum is added to a suspension of cephalin and cholesterol. The extent of flocculation is observed at the end of 24 and 48 hours.

Possible interfering materials and conditions Both false positive and false negative reactions may occur if the patient is taking methyldopa (Aldomet, Aldoril).

Normal range *Adults:* Either negative or 1+. Reports are delayed 24 to 48 hours. *Children:* This test is not considered reliable in children.

Ceruloplasmin

This enzyme is active in copper transport. Measurement of blood levels of ceruloplasmin is useful in diagnosing hepatolenticular degeneration (Wilson's disease), in which levels of this enzyme are depressed. Ceruloplasmin levels are elevated in several other conditions including leukemia, Hodgkins' disease, hyperthyroidism, cirrhosis, and myocardial infarction. However, because of the wide variety of conditions associated with increased ceruloplasmin levels, a higher than normal level of the enzyme is of little diagnostic value.

Food and drink restrictions None.

Procedure for collecting specimen Collect at least 3 ml of *venous* blood in a collecting tube with a red stopper.

Laboratory procedure   The rate at which the sample containing ceruloplasmin oxidizes an indicator substance is measured either spectrophotometrically or photometrically.

Possible interfering materials and conditions   None reported yet.

Normal range   *Adults:* 20-35 mg/100 ml. *Infants under 6 months:* Levels under 20 mg/100 ml may be normal and do not indicate the presence of any disease.

Chlorides

Chlorides are measured to help diagnose disorders in the maintenance of normal osmotic relationships, acid-base balance, and water balance of the body. Usually this test is performed together with measurement of other ions of the blood.

An elevation in blood chlorides (hyperchloremia) occurs in several conditions, including various kidney disorders, Cushing's syndrome, and hyperventilation. A decrease in blood chlorides (hypochloremia) is seen in such states as excessive vomiting and diarrhea, diabetic acidosis, Addison's disease, and heat exhaustion, and following certain surgical procedures.

Food and drink restrictions   None.

Procedure for collecting specimen   Collect 5 ml of *venous* blood in a collecting tube with a red stopper.

Laboratory procedure   In many laboratories, a chloridometer is used.

Possible interfering materials and conditions   There may be an apparent elevation of chloride if the patient has been taking bromides (Fello-Sed, Neurosine).

Normal range   *Adults:* 95 to 106 mEq/L of serum. *Children:* Similar to adult levels. This, however, depends on the laboratory method used.

Cholesterol

Cholesterol is a normal constituent of the blood and is found in all cells, but its exact physiologic function is not clear. It may serve as the substance from which various hormones are synthesized. In various disease states the cholesterol concentration in the serum may be raised or lowered. Cholesterol levels are elevated in many conditions; in most the finding is only incidental. An elevated cholesterol level may be helpful in the diagnosis of xanthomatosis, certain liver diseases, and hypothyroidism. There is also increasing interest in the role of cholesterol in producing myocardial infarction, since deposits of cholesterol, known as plaques, are often found partially blocking the coronary arteries. However, there is as yet no conclusive evidence linking this condition to the blood serum cholesterol concentration. Decreased serum cholesterol is found in hyperthyroidism, anemias, starvation, and acute infections.

Food and drink restrictions   Serum cholesterol levels are not influenced by diet over a short period of time, although they are affected over a long period of time. Therefore, fasting is *not* required before taking the sample. However, it would probably be prudent to avoid foods containing large amounts of cholesterol for the 12 hours preceding the test. Such foods are egg yolk and brains. On the other hand, some laboratories do triglyceride levels at the same time and require a 12- to 14-hour fast. It is advisable to check with the laboratory.

Procedure for collecting specimen   Collect 5 ml of *venous* blood in a collecting tube with a red stopper.

Laboratory procedure   Several procedures are available. A direct colorimetric method is becoming widely used.

Possible interfering materials and conditions   The cholesterol level may be spuriously elevated if the patient has taken any of the following: bile salts, bromides, metandienone, vitamin A.

Another drug, diphenylhydantoin (Dilantin), may also elevate cholesterol levels, but it is not known whether this is an interference or a pharmacologic effect.

Certain antibiotics, notably the tetracyclines and neomycin, may produce a true, but temporary and misleading, reduction in cholesterol levels.

Anoxia may increase serum cholesterol levels.

Hemolysis may produce a spurious elevation of cholesterol levels.

Normal range   Expressed in milligrams per 100 milliliters of serum (mg/100 ml), as listed below:

Adults: 120 to 260

Many persons over the age of 30 have cholesterol levels that are higher than 260 mg/100 ml. It has been suggested that the upper limit of normal be considered about 360 mg/100 ml. We do not know whether the higher levels in people over 30 are truly normal, physiological, and harmless, or whether substantial numbers of these people already have atherosclerosis, and that this is reflected in the cholesterol level. It will take years to resolve this problem in interpretation.

Children: Newborn: 50 to 100

1 week to 1 year: 70 to 175

1 year to adolescence: 135 to 240

Cholesterol Esters

This liver function test is being phased out since it is much less specific than other tests now available.

Clotting (Coagulation) Time

This test measures the ability of blood to clot. Many factors are involved in clotting, including prothrombin, thromboplastin, and fibrinogen. New clotting factors are continually being discovered. A deficiency of any essential factor or an increase in inhibitory factors may prolong clotting time. This test is distinct from the bleeding time test since the latter also involves the ability of small blood vessels to constrict. This test, furthermore, should not be confused with special clotting time measurements that use siliconized or lusteroid test tubes.

Food and drink restrictions   None.

Procedure for performing test and collecting specimen   There are several methods. The most common ones involve the use of venous blood. Freshly drawn blood is put into 4 small test tubes (1 ml in each) and the first tube is tilted at 30-second intervals. When clotting is observed, the same procedure is followed in succession with the other 3 tubes. The clotting time is the average of the times elapsed between venipuncture and clotting in the last 3 tubes.

Possible interfering materials and conditions None reported yet.

Normal range *Adults: By this method,* 5 to 8 minutes according to some authorities; 6 to 17 minutes according to others. *Children:* Similar to the range for adults.

CO_2 Combining Power

This test is gradually being replaced by other tests of carbon dioxide and electrolytes. However, because it is relatively simple, it is still useful. The test is a general measure of the acidity or alkalinity of the blood. An increase in CO_2 combining power is usually a manifestation of alkalosis, while a decrease is usually a manifestation of acidosis. However, changes in CO_2 combining power do not always represent changes in pH of the blood, since the latter depends on the ratio, not on the absolute amounts, of basic and acidic substances. As in many other tests, good clinical judgment is needed to evaluate the results. High CO_2 combining power is usually found in conditions such as persistent vomiting or drainage of the stomach with loss of hydrochloric acid, excessive intake of sodium bicarbonate in the presence of poor kidney function, excessive administration of ACTH or cortisone, and hypoventilation. Low CO_2 combining power is usually found in such conditions as diabetic acidosis, severe diarrhea or drainage of intestinal fluids, certain kidney diseases, and hyperventilation. In many cases it is also necessary to test the pH of the blood to evaluate properly the acid-base balance. The CO_2 combining power test may, in some situations, be designated by the physician as "emergency."

Food and drink restrictions None.

Procedure for collecting specimen Using a collecting tube with a green stopper, collect *venous* blood without using a tourniquet, if possible. If a tourniquet is necessary, the patient should *not* open and close his fist, but should keep it closed without straining. For years, the blood sample was collected under oil. However, there is a growing trend away from this practice. Instead, vacuum tubes containing heparin are used, and 7 ml of blood collected in them. In some hospitals, oiled syringes are still used, and can give satisfactory results.

Laboratory procedure   Usually the Van Slyke apparatus is used. The serum sample is equilibrated with alveolar air. Then the carbon dioxide, combined with the serum, is freed by adding an acid, and the volume is measured.

Possible interfering materials and conditions   The carbon dioxide combining power may be spuriously decreased if the patient has taken nitrofurantoin.

Normal range   *Adults:* 24 to 35 mEq/L. *Children:* This test is no longer done commonly on children. Instead, carbon dioxide levels (see p. 48) are determined.

Coagulation   *See* Clotting Time

Cold Agglutinins

This is a test for atypical viral pneumonia. Almost everyone has agglutinins that will cause agglutination of his or her own red cells at refrigerator temperatures. However, this ordinarily occurs when the serum is not diluted, or only moderately diluted. In viral pneumonia, the cold agglutinins increase in titer and cause agglutination even at relatively high dilutions.

Food and drink restrictions   None.

Procedure for collecting specimen   Collect 7 ml of *venous* blood in a collecting tube with a red stopper. The specimen must be kept near body temperature; *it must not be refrigerated*. It should be sent to the laboratory at once.

Laboratory procedure   A serial tube dilution method is used, with incubation in a refrigerator overnight.

Possible interfering materials and conditions   Refrigeration of blood sample before separation of serum.

Normal range   *Adults:* A titer less than 1:16. Some laboratories use 1:32. *Children:* No differences from the range for adults have been established.

Congo Red Retention

This test is no longer in common use.

Coombs' Direct

This is also called a direct antiglobulin test. It is a basic immunologic procedure that reveals antigen-antibody reactions that are, in a sense, incomplete or weak. For example, antibodies to human red cells may combine with the red cells in such a way as to damage them, or increase their fragility but not cause visible agglutination. Such antibodies are demonstrated by Coombs' test. It may be used in a wide variety of clinical or microbiological applications. Its major clinical uses, however, are in the early diagnosis of erythroblastosis fetalis and autoimmune hemolytic anemia. A positive direct Coombs' test indicates that some antibody is attached to the red cells, but does not indicate the exact nature of the antibody. Many different diseases may produce a positive direct Coombs'.

Food and drink restrictions None.

Procedure for collecting specimen Fresh clotted blood is considered superior by several authorities. Venous blood may be used or, in the case of newborns, blood from the umbilical cord. Usually 2 ml of blood is sufficient; it should be collected in a collecting tube with a red stopper.

Laboratory procedure A washed suspension of the patient's red blood cells is added to some Coombs' serum (rabbit anti-human globulin) purchased from a reliable biological supply house. The red cells are then observed for agglutination. Results may be reported as 1 + to 4 +.

Possible interfering materials and conditions Many drugs can produce a positive direct Coombs' reaction. It is not clear whether this is an interference or a pharmacologic effect. The drugs, listed by official (generic) name include: aminopyrine, cephaloridine, cephalothin (effect may persist for months), methyldopa (effect may persist for months), penicillin (effect may persist for months).

Heparin may interfere in cases of acquired hemolytic anemia and produce a negative direct Coombs'.

Normal range *Adults:* Normally the direct Coombs' test is negative. *Children:* Same as for adults.

Coombs' Indirect

The indirect Coombs' test is used in detection of the various minor blood type factors, including Rh. If red cells of known antigenic composition (i.e., the minor blood type factors) are used, the related antibody content of a test serum can be determined. The reverse procedure may also be used. In cross-matching blood for transfusions, this test may be used to eliminate bloods that might cause reactions because of incompatibilities of the minor blood type factors.

Food and drink restrictions None.

Procedure for collecting specimen Fresh clotted blood is considered superior by several authorities. Usually 5 ml of blood is sufficient; it should be collected in a collecting tube with a red stopper.

Laboratory procedure Donor red cells and recipient serum are mixed together and allowed to stand. Then the red cells are removed, washed, and antiglobulin is added. The reaction may be reported from 1 + to 4 +.

Possible interfering materials and conditions None reported yet.

Normal range *Adults:* Usually the test is negative. *Children:* Same as for adults.

Cortisol

Cortisol, also known as hydrocortisone or Compound F, is the major secretion of the adrenal cortex. The plasma cortisol levels are low in androgenital syndrome and Addison's disease. Elevations are sometimes found in Cushing's syndrome, extreme stress, eclampsia, acute pancreatitis, extensive surgery, and burns.

Food and drink restrictions None reported.

Procedure for collecting specimen   Collect 5 to 10 ml of *venous* blood in a collecting tube with a stopper of the color specified by the laboratory. The amount required varies from laboratory to laboratory, as does the color of the stopper of the collecting tube.

Laboratory procedure   Several procedures are available and vary from laboratory to laboratory.

Possible interfering materials and conditions   Spironolactone, triparanol, and oral contraceptives may produce a spuriously high level.

Normal range   Expressed in micrograms per 100 milliliters (mcg/100 ml).

Adults: 8 a.m.: 5 to 27
4 p.m.: 2 to 18
These figures vary considerably between hospital laboratories.

Children: This test is not ordinarily performed on children, and the normal range is not definitely established.

CPK   *See* Creatine Phosphokinase

C-Reactive Protein (CRP)

This test for inflammation and tissue breakdown is being used less frequently than in the past. It is nonspecific and similar to the sedimentation rate test. The C-reactive protein test is positive in myocardial infarction, acute rheumatic fever, widespread cancer, malaria, bacterial infection, and other conditions. It is sometimes used to follow the activity of a disease. The term C-reactive protein was chosen because the protein involved forms a precipitate with the C-polysaccharide of the pneumococcus. The relationship between this action and its use in diagnosis is not clear, and the clinical use of the test is based on the empirical observation that it is positive in conditions with widespread inflammation and tissue breakdown.

Food and drink restrictions   None.

Procedure for collecting specimen   Collect 5 ml of *venous* blood in a collecting tube with a red stopper.

Laboratory procedure   A sample of the serum is mixed with C-reactive protein antiserum. If a precipitate forms, the test is positive.

Possible interfering materials and conditions   None reported yet.

Normal range   *Adults:* No C-reactive protein is present in the blood. *Children:* Same as for adults.

Creatine Phosphokinase (CPK)

This test is useful in the diagnosis of two quite different diseases, myocardial infarction and muscular dystrophy. The enzyme is found in both cardiac and skeletal muscle. In myocardial infarction, the rise in serum creatine phosphokinase may start in about four hours, and in 24 to 36 hours reach a peak at which the levels may be 50 to 100 times the normal levels. In early muscular dystrophy, often before clinical signs are clear, the creatine phosphokinase levels may be 300 to 400 times normal.

Food and drink restrictions   None reported yet.

Procedure for collecting specimen   Collect 5 ml of *venous* blood in a collecting tube with a red stopper.

Laboratory procedure   Several different methods of measuring creatine phosphokinase levels are available. All of them measure the activity of the enzyme.

Possible interfering materials and conditions   Severe exercise may produce moderate increases in creatine phosphokinase levels, but not usually enough to mimic the serious diseases for which the test is used. Any condition causing severe muscle destruction, such as crush syndrome, may result in high levels. Slight elevations occur in dermatomyositis, delirium tremens, and hypothyroidism.

For reasons that are still unclear, some cases of pulmonary infarction and pulmonary edema may have high creatine phosphokinase levels.

Electrocautery used within the preceding few days may also produce elevated levels.

Slight muscle injury, such as that produced by intramuscular injections, can also elevate the creatine phosphokinase.

Normal range

Adults: This may be expressed in several ways, depending on the method of assay used and the laboratory. Thus one must know the range considered normal by the laboratory doing the measurement. Examples of normal ranges are:

> 1 to 12 Sigma units/ml
> 0 to 100 MU/ml
> 5 to 50 U/ml
> 1 to 12 IU/L

Children: Newborns tend to have higher levels that later drop. The normal range depends on the laboratory and the technique used.

Creatinine

This test is a measurement of kidney function similar to the urea nitrogen test. Creatinine is derived from the breakdown of muscle creatine phosphate. The amount produced per day is relatively constant, and it is excreted by the kidney. An elevated blood creatinine level indicates a disorder of kidney function.

Food and drink restrictions   None.

Procedure for collecting specimen   Collect 5 ml of *venous* blood in a collecting tube with a red stopper.

Laboratory procedure   Alkaline picrate is added to the serum sample. The color produced is compared to standards and the concentration of creatinine calculated.

Possible interfering materials and conditions   A spuriously high level of serum creatinine may result if the patient has had either a BSP (Bromsulphalein) or PSP (phenolsulfonphthalein) test within the previous 24 hours.

In addition, several drugs can produce spuriously high levels. The drugs, listed by generic name, include: ascorbic acid, barbiturates, and chlordiazepoxide.

Spuriously low levels may be produced by methyldopa.

Normal range   *Adults:* 0.6 to 1.3 mg/100 ml. *Children:* 0.4 to 1.2 mg/100 ml.

Cryoglobulins

Cryoglobulins are serum globulins that precipitate at about 4°C and redissolve when warmed. They are not normally present, but are found in many pathologic conditions including systemic lupus erythematosus, leukemia, multiple myeloma, rheumatoid arthritis, and others. The value of a cryoglobulin determination is not yet clear, but perhaps in the future more will be learned from it.

Food and drink restrictions None.

Procedure for collecting specimen Collect *venous* blood in a collecting tube with a red stopper. For qualitative tests, 3 ml are needed. For quantitative tests, 10 ml are needed. The specimen must not be refrigerated before being delivered to the laboratory.

Laboratory procedure The serum is cooled to 4°C and the presence or absence of a precipitate observed.

Possible interfering materials and conditions None reported yet.

Normal range *Adults:* No cryoglobulins are present in the blood. *Children:* Same as for adults.

CT *See* Clotting Time

Culture *See* Blood Culture, Chapter 2

Differential Count *See* Blood Counts, White Cell Differential Count

Digitoxin

This test is basically similar to the test for digoxin. However, the safe level of digitoxin is substantially higher. The nontoxic levels of digitoxin are generally less than 18 ng/ml (nanogram/milliliter).

Digoxin

The level of digoxin in the serum is directly related to therapeutic effect and toxicity. Proper levels of digoxin, a cardiac glycoside, increase the force of the heart beat in congestive heart failure.

Excessive levels, however, produce many kinds of toxicity, including arrhythmias and death. Before a reliable test for digoxin levels was developed, the cardiac glycosides were responsible for many deaths. The availability of this test has greatly reduced mortality and serious toxicity resulting from use of digoxin. It has also made underdosage less likely.

Food and drink restrictions None.

Procedure for collecting specimen Collect 5 ml of *venous* blood in a collecting tube with a red stopper. The spelling of the drug whose level is sought *must* be carefully checked, since different antibodies are used for digoxin and digitoxin.

Laboratory procedure A radioimmunoassay procedure is most widely used.

Possible interfering materials and conditions None reported yet.

Normal range *Adults:* Normally, there is no digoxin in the serum. If the patient is being treated with digoxin, levels below 2 ng/ml (nanogram/milliliter) are not usually toxic, while levels over 2 ng/ml are likely to be toxic. *Children:* Some infants may tolerate digoxin levels slightly over 2 ng/ml but, in general, it seems prudent to try to keep the levels just under or at 2 ng/ml.

Dilantin *See* Diphenylhydantoin

Diphenylhydantoin (Dilantin)

The serum levels of diphenylhydantoin are measured in order to adjust the dosage of this antiepileptic drug. At times, diphenylhydantoin is also used in the treatment of cardiac arrhythmias, and here too knowledge of serum levels is helpful in adjusting dosage.

Food and drink restrictions None.

Procedure for collecting specimen Collect 5 ml of *venous* blood in a collecting tube with a red stopper.

Laboratory procedure Several procedures are available. Gas-liquid chromatography is considered the method of choice when it is available.

Possible interfering materials and conditions None.

Normal range *Adults:* In the absence of treatment, there is no diphenylhydantoin in the serum. Therapeutic levels for the treatment of epilepsy range from 15 to 20 mcg/ml. Therapeutic levels for the treatment of cardiac arrhythmias are 10 to 18 mcg/ml. Mild to moderate toxicity may occur at levels of 30 to 40 mcg/ml. At about 40 mcg/ml, serious toxicity is likely. In general, each patient must have a base line recorded in order to assess the significance of the diphenylhydantoin levels. *Children:* At times, children may require slightly higher therapeutic concentrations than adults, but exact levels have not yet been established.

Doriden   *See* Glutethimide

Erythrocyte Count   *See* Blood Counts, Red Cell Count

ESR   *See* Sedimentation Rate

Fasting Blood Sugar (FBS)   *See* Glucose (Sugar)

Fibrinogen

In conditions characterized by inadequate blood clotting it may be helpful to determine which element of the clotting mechanism is deficient. The fibrinogen of the plasma is essential for blood clotting. In the presence of thrombin it is converted to insoluble fibrin threads. Measurement of the blood fibrinogen level may aid in establishing the cause of a clotting deficiency.

Food and drink restrictions   None.

Procedure for collecting specimen   Collect *venous* blood in a collecting tube with a blue or orange stopper, depending on the laboratory. The full capacity of the tube should be used.

Laboratory procedure   Several procedures are now available. One commonly used is a colorimetric measurement of the tyrosine in the fibrinogen.

Possible interfering materials and conditions   None reported yet.

Normal range   200 to 600 mg/100 ml of plasma. Plasma normally contains more fibrinogen than is actually needed for satisfactory clotting. Deficiencies in blood clotting due to fibrinogen deficiency do not occur until the concentration falls to 75 mg/100 ml of plasma.

Folic Acid

This test is performed to help diagnose folic acid deficiency. In pregnancy, the fetal requirement for folic acid is so great that sometimes the mother develops a folic acid deficiency. In other conditions associated with intestinal malabsorption and or inadequate utilization of folic acid, folic acid deficiency marked by megaloblastic anemia may occur.

Food and drink restrictions   None.

Procedure for collecting specimen   Collect 7 ml of *venous* blood in a collecting tube with a red stopper.

Laboratory procedure   Originally, a microbiologic assay was used. A radioisotope assay is also available.

Possible interfering materials and conditions   None reported yet.

Normal range   *Adults:* 7 to 16 ng/ml (nanogram/milliliter) in some hospital laboratories, 4 to 20 ng/ml in others, depending on procedure used. *Children:* This test is not ordinarily performed on children and normal values have not been established.

Fragility, Osmotic   *See* Red Cell Fragility

FTA-ABS   *See* Fluorescent Treponemal Antibody Absorption

Gammopathies   *See* Plasma Electrophoresis for Gammopathies

Globulin   *See* Albumin, Globulin, Total Protein, A/G Ratio

Glucose (Sugar)

This test is performed to discover whether there is a disorder of glucose metabolism. An increase in blood glucose level is found in severe diabetes, chronic liver disease, and overactivity of several of the endocrine glands. A symptom caused directly by the elevated blood sugar is occasional, intermittent blurring of vision. In mild diabetes there may be a normal glucose level so that more sensitive tests need to be performed (*see* Glucose Tolerance). There may be a decrease in blood sugar in persons with tumors of the islets of Langerhans in the pancreas, underfunctioning of various endocrine glands, glycogen storage disease (von Gierke's), and overtreatment with insulin. If the blood glucose level falls too low, coma, convulsions, and even death may result.

Food and drink restrictions   The patient must fast for 12 hours before the test. Water is permitted.

Procedure for collecting specimen   Collect 5 ml of *venous* blood in a collecting tube with a gray stopper.

Laboratory procedure   Several procedures are available. Most laboratories now use an automated method.

Possible interfering materials and conditions   The blood glucose levels may be high if the patient has taken ACTH, physostigmine, or an overdose of nalidixic acid (Neg Gram).

If the o-toluidine method is used to measure glucose, the administration of dextrans to the patient may give spuriously high levels.

Normal range   Expressed in milligrams per 100 milliliters (mg/100 ml) of either serum *or* whole blood, as listed below.

Adults: 80 to 120 (serum) *or*
70 to 105 (whole blood)
The values above will be obtained if one of the older laboratory procedures is used. With some newer procedures, normal range may be:
70 to 110 (serum) *or*
60 to 95 (whole blood)

Children: Newborn: 20 to 80 (whole blood)
Others: Blood glucose levels rise rapidly to adult levels within a few weeks or months after birth.

Glucose-6-phosphate Dehydrogenase Test (G6PD)

This is a test for congenital deficiency of an enzyme, glucose-6-phosphate dehydrogenase, in the red blood cells. Acute hemolytic anemia may develop in patients with such a deficiency when certain drugs (such as primaquine) or foods (such as fava beans) are taken. A knowledge of the existence of this congenital deficiency can be helpful in advising the patient about avoidance of substances that can precipitate hemolytic anemia, and also for genetic counseling.

Food and drink restrictions   None.

Procedure for collecting specimen   Several are available. One requires the collection of a small amount of capillary blood in a heparinized microhematocrit tube. Another requires the collection of 4 ml of *venous* blood in a collecting tube with a stopper of the appropriate color. The laboratory of each institution should be asked which collection procedure it requires.

Laboratory procedure   Several different laboratory procedures are available.

Possible interfering materials and conditions   None reported yet.

Normal range   Normally, the tests show substantial amounts (by color or staining techniques) of glucose-6-phosphate dehydrogenase in the red cells.

Glucose Tolerance

These tests are used to discover disorders of glucose metabolism that have not become severe enough to change the blood glucose levels in the fasting state. In the glucose tolerance tests, a large amount of glucose is given to a fasting patient, either intravenously or orally. At regular intervals thereafter, the blood glucose levels are measured to learn how long it takes the body to handle the added glucose. If it remains in the blood for an excessive period of time, there is some disorder of carbohydrate metabolism. The intravenous test is somewhat more sensitive than the oral, since the factor of absorption from the gastrointestinal tract is not involved. In the oral test, an increase in blood sugar and its persistence for 3 hours is seen in diabetes. In the intravenous test the blood sugar is, of course, elevated in all cases. If the blood glucose concentration does not return to normal within less than 3 hours after the intravenous administration of glucose, diabetes is probably present. If 1 to 2 hours are required to return to normal there may be some liver disorder. The urine voided during the course of this test is examined for sugar to obtain additional information about the kidney excretion of excess sugar.

Food and drink restrictions The patient should be on an adequate diet, containing at least 150 gm of carbohydrate per day for at least one week. For 12 hours before the test, the patient must fast, but may have water ad lib.

Procedures for collecting specimen Procedures differ in various laboratories. One procedure is as follows:

1. Collect 2 to 3 ml of *venous* blood in a collecting tube with a gray or a red stopper, depending on the color specified by the laboratory.
2. Collect urine specimen at once.
3. If the intravenous test is used the doctor will administer intravenously by slow infusion 0.5 gm of glucose/kg of body weight. He will use a 20% solution and take 30 minutes for the infusion.
3a. If the oral test is used, the patient receives 1.75 gm of glucose/kg of body weight in unsweetened lemonade. Commercial preparations containing the appropriate amounts of glucose in beverages or gels are also available.
4. If the intravenous test is used, 2 to 3 ml of *venous* blood are collected immediately from the arm that did not receive the infusion. Subsequent withdrawals of blood are made exactly 30, 60, 90, and 150 minutes after the infusion. Each time a sample is collected, a urine specimen is also collected.
4a. In the oral test, 2 to 3 ml of *venous* blood are collected 30, 60, 120, and 180 minutes after ingestion of the glucose. Each time a sample is collected, a urine specimen is also collected.
5. Each specimen must be labeled with the date and time of collection.

Laboratory procedure The laboratory will test each blood sample as described under Glucose and each urine sample as described under Sugar, Qualitative (Chapter 5).

Possible interfering materials and conditions The glucose tolerance curve may be altered if the patient has taken any of the following: isocarboxazid, oral contraceptives, phenelzine.

Normal range *Adults:* Oral: Peak of not more than 150 mg/100 ml or serum; return to fasting level within 2 hours. Intravenous: Return to fasting level within about 1 hour.

Recent evidence suggests that the above criteria may be much too strict for middle-aged and elderly subjects. In a reappraisal, West considers that for patients over 59 years of age, one hour values as high as 200 mg/100 ml may be within normal limits. *Children:* This depends on the child's age and the particular laboratory.

Glycosides, Cardiac *See* Digoxin

G6PD *See* Glucose-6-phosphate Dehydrogenase Test

Grouping *See* Blood Types

GT *See* Glucose Tolerance

GTT *See* Glucose Tolerance Test

Guthrie

This is a blood test for the presence of phenylketonuria. It is used as a general screening procedure for young infants before they leave the hospital. It is useful on infants as young as three days, although it can be performed on older infants also. The Guthrie test has one advantage over the urine test for phenylketonuria (see p. 162). The urine test is not ordinarily significant until the age of three weeks, and by that time the infant has usually left the hospital.

A negative Guthrie test means that there is no appreciable danger of phenylketonuria. A positive test does not definitely establish phenylketonuria, but means that there is a considerable chance of its being present. If the Guthrie test is positive, a more intricate test-measurement of blood phenylalanine levels is ordinarily necessary. However, this is not usually done in the average hospital laboratory, but in specially equipped laboratories.

The Guthrie test is one of the legally acceptable tests for phenylketonuria in states that require testing of all newborns for the disease.

Food and drink restrictions   None.

Procedure for collecting specimen   The heel of the infant is pricked with a disposable lancet and three drops of blood are collected on a piece of special filter paper furnished by the laboratory.

The blood specimen must be collected no earlier than the third day of life, and no earlier than 48 hours after the start of feeding with milk or protein-containing substitute.

Laboratory procedure   The filter paper is autoclaved and a small circle punched from the center of a bloodstain. This small punch-out is then placed on the surface of a Petri dish containing nutrient agar mixed with a substrate that inhibits Bacillus subtilis, and the surface is then well streaked with a culture of that bacillus. If the bacillus does not grow near the blood-stained filter paper, the test is negative. If the bacillus does grow near the filter paper, the test is positive.

Possible interfering materials and conditions   None reported yet.

Normal range   Usually the Guthrie test is negative.

HAA (Hepatitis Associated Antigen)   *See* Australia Antigen Assay

Haptoglobin

This is a test for hemolysis. Haptoglobins are globulin molecules with a particular affinity for free hemoglobin that may be liberated when red blood cells are destroyed within blood vessels. The combination of haptoglobin and hemoglobin is fairly firm. In cases of red blood cell destruction (hemolysis), much of the haptoglobin is bound to the hemoglobin, so that the level of free haptoglobin is decreased. Therefore, a lower than normal haptoglobin level suggests hemolysis. In a small proportion of persons, there is a congenital absence of haptoglobin and, in these cases, the low level does not seem to be associated with disease. Haptoglobin levels are also decreased in some severe liver disorders and in infectious mononucleosis.

An increase in haptoglobin levels may occur in an inflammatory disease or during steroid therapy. This is not, in itself, of diagnostic significance. However, it can mask a hemolytic process.

Food and drink restrictions   None.

Procedure for collecting specimen   Collect 5 ml of *venous* blood in a collecting tube with a red stopper.

Laboratory procedure   Several procedures are available, both electrophoretic and spectrophotometric.

Possible interfering materials and conditions   An elevation in free haptoglobin levels, masking a hemolytic condition, may occur if the patient has been on steroid therapy recently, or has an inflammation.

Normal range   *Adults:* 100 to 200 mg/100 ml. *Children:* This varies with age. At birth, most infants have no measurable serum haptoglobin. From the age of 1 month, levels begin to rise, reaching about 30 mg/100 ml at 6 months. Then there is a slower rise toward adult levels. The test is of virtually no value for diagnosing hemolysis in infants and young children.

Hb   *See* Hemoglobin

Heat-Stable Lactic Dehydrogenase (HLDH)

This is becoming less commonly used. It is primarily an aid in the diagnosis of myocardial infarction in cases in which the regular lactic dehydrogenase test may not be sufficiently specific. Lactic dehydrogenase, of which at least 5 different types are known, is found in serum and in several organs. Thus, an elevated level of lactic dehydrogenase might result from a variety of conditions (p. 82). It has been found that one type of lactic dehydrogenase is stable when heated in a particular manner and that it is more specific in cases of myocardial infarction than are the others. Consequently, when the diagnosis is in doubt, a heat-stable lactic dehydrogenase test may be done.

Food and drink restrictions   None reported.

Procedure for collecting specimen   Collect 3 to 5 ml of *venous* blood in a collecting tube with a red stopper.

Laboratory procedure A specimen of the serum is kept at a fixed, elevated temperature for a fixed period of time. Then the enzyme activity is measured as described under lactic dehydrogenase.

Possible interfering materials and conditions If any oxalate comes in contact with the specimen, it will cause falsely low readings. Megaloblastic anemia, hemolytic anemia, and muscular dystrophy may produce false positive results.

Normal range *Adults:* The normal range is not precisely known. In general, experts consider values below 115 units not clearly diagnostic of myocardial infarction, while values over 115 units generally are. *Children:* This test is not ordinarily performed on children.

Hgb *See* Hemoglobin

Hematocrit

This test measures the relative volume of cells and plasma in the blood. In anemias and after hemorrhage the hematocrit reading is lowered; in polycythmia and dehydration it is raised.

Food and drink restrictions None.

Procedure for collecting specimen Collect *venous* blood in a collecting tube with a lavender stopper. The tube must be filled.

Laboratory procedure The blood is carefully placed in a special (Wintrobe) tube up to the 0 mark. The tube is then spun in a centrifuge and the height of the column of packed red blood cells measured against the graduations on the side of the tube.

Possible interfering materials and conditions None reported yet.

Normal range Expressed in millimeters per 100 millimeters (mm/100 mm) of column height, or as the percentage, which is the same figure (that is, 50 mm/100 mm is the same as 50%).

Adults: Men: 40 to 50
         Women: 35 to 45

Children: Newborn to 1 month: 42 to 54
          1 month to 3 months: 29 to 54

    3 months to 12 months: 29 to 41
    1 year to 3 years: 29 to 40
    3 years to 10 years: 36 to 38

Hemoglobin

Hemoglobin, the essential oxygen carrier of the blood, is found within the red blood cells and is responsible for the red color of the blood. The hemoglobin is decreased in hemorrhage and anemias and increased in hemoconcentration and polycythemia. The hemoglobin and red cell count do not always rise or fall equally. This fact is often important in differential diagnosis of anemias. In iron deficiency (microcytic) anemia, hemoglobin is reduced more than the red blood cell count. In pernicious anemia, the red cell count is reduced more than hemoglobin.

Food and drink restrictions None.

Procedure for collecting specimen Ordinarily, *capillary* blood is obtained from a fingerprick and a tiny amount taken into the appropriate pipette. However, sometimes *venous* blood is collected in a vacuum tube. If so, the tube must be filled. If venous blood is used, the color of the collecting tube stopper should be lavender.

Laboratory procedure Usually a spectrophotometric technique is used.

Normal range Expressed in grams per 100 milliliters (gm/100 ml) of blood.

   Adults: 12 to 18

   Children: Newborn to 1 month: 14 to 19.5
                 10 months to 1 year: 11.2 to 14
                 1 year to 3 years: 11.2 to 12.5
                 3 years to 10 years: 12.5 to 13

Hemoglobin Electrophoresis

This is a test to identify abnormal hemoglobins. There are at least 150 different hemoglobins, most of them differing from the common hemoglobin only by a single amino acid. These abnormal hemoglobins are genetically transmitted and a patient may have two of them, one from each parent. Not all of them produce clinical symptoms. The most common one (Hb S), produces sickling (p. 112). The most common clinical sign of the presence of abnormal hemoglobins is anemia that is resistant to ordinary treatment. The hemoglobins are designated by a series of letters, numbers, and subscripts that are related to their mobility during electrophoresis and to where they were discovered. Normal hemoglobin is hemoglobin A (Hb A). Abnormal hemoglobins are Hb D, Hb E, Hb A_2, Hb M_{Boston}, and so forth.

Food and drink restrictions   None.

Procedure for collecting specimen   The patient should not have had a blood transfusion during the preceding four months. Collect *venous* blood in a collecting tube with a lavender stopper. The tube should be filled.

Laboratory procedure   The red cells are washed and then hemolysed. The hemolysed material is subjected to electrophoresis and the bands compared to known standards.

Possible interfering materials and conditions   A blood transfusion given during the preceding four months may cause the results to be spurious.

Normal range   Normally, only hemoglobin A is present in adults. In infants, hemoglobin F is also present until the age of about two years.

Hepatitis Test   *See* Australia Antigen Assay

Heterophile Antibody

This is a test for infectious mononucleosis. In this disease, the level (titer) of antibodies to sheep erythrocytes rises for reasons that are not known. If the antibody level rises so that agglutination of sheep erythrocytes occurs at dilutions of 1:112 or greater, the test is considered positive. However, there are sometimes other antisheep erythrocyte antibodies in the blood, that are not related to infectious mononucleosis. Accordingly, it may be necessary to repeat the test by using more complicated techniques of antibody absorption.

Food and drink restrictions   None.

Procedure for collecting specimen   Collect 5 ml of *venous* blood in a collecting tube with a red stopper.

Laboratory procedure Serial dilutions of the patient's serum are added to washed suspensions of sheep erythrocytes in a series of test tubes and incubated. The greatest dilution that agglutinates the erythrocytes is noted.

A rapid slide test that gives results in a few minutes is now available for office use.

Possible interfering materials and conditions None reported yet.

Normal range Agglutination in concentrations up to 1:28.

Hinton *See* Serological Tests for Syphilis

HLDH *See* Heat-Stable Lactic Dehydrogenase

IBC *See* Iron Binding Capacity

Icterus Index

This is a measure of the degree of yellowness of the serum. It is a way to determine whether there is excess bilirubin (bile pigment) in the serum. This test is being phased out and, instead, many institutions are using the more specific bilirubin measurement (p. 36).

IGA *See* Immunoglobulins

IGG *See* Immunoglobulins

IGM *See* Immunoglobulins

II *See* Icterus Index

Immunoglobulins (Ig)

Immunoglobulins are a type of protein found in the gamma globulin fraction of serum. They comprise the major antibodies. The immunoglobulins have been fractionated into five main fractions: immunoglobulin A (IgA), immunoglobulin D (IgD), immunoglobulin E (IgE), immunoglobulin G (IgG), and immunoglobulin M (IgM).

The most important ones at this time seem to be A, G, and M, although this may change with further research. In recent years, many studies have been done on the quantitative alterations in the various immunoglobulin fractions in different disease states. This research is continuing at a fast pace, and new developments are to be expected. Thus far, it has been shown that a wide variety of diseases are associated with changes in the levels of one or more immunoglobulin fractions. These diseases include agammaglobulinemia, acute leukemias, ataxia-telangiectasia, biliary cirrhosis, chronic leukemias, dysgammaglobulinemia, Hodgkin's disease, Laennec's cirrhosis, lymphoid aplasia, macroglobulinemia, nephrotic syndrome, rheumatoid arthritis, systemic lupus erythematosus, tuberculosis, and trypanosomiasis. We can expect other disorders to be added to this list. The pattern of quantitative change in the immunoglobulin fractions varies in a complex way depending on the disorder. It is not practical to attempt to describe in this book all the patterns that exist. An expert clinical immunologist should interpret the findings. This test appears to have the potential of an excellent diagnostic tool, and advances in its use may be expected soon.

Food and drink restrictions None.

Procedure for collecting specimen Collect 5 to 10 ml of *venous* blood in a collecting tube with a red stopper.

Laboratory procedure The technique of radial immunodiffusion is used.

Possible interfering materials and conditions Passive antisera (such as gamma globulin and tetanus antitoxin), blood transfusions, and transfusion of blood components will produce confusing results for a variable time. Active immunization, such as the use of toxoids, may also confuse the findings and, if the patient has had such immunization in the previous 6 months, it should be reported to the laboratory and noted on the chart.

Normal range Expressed in milligrams per 100 milliliters (mg/100 ml). Typical values vary among hospital laboratories; the figures below come from one major hospital laboratory.

Adults: IgA: 160-400
         IgG: 800-1500
         IgM: 50-110

Children: The newborn levels are close to those of adults for IgG, but much lower for IgA and IgM. By the age of 6 weeks, the IgG level has fallen to one-fourth or one-third the adult level, and the IgA and IgM levels are rising slowly. Thereafter, all levels rise gradually until adulthood.

Insulin Tolerance

This test is no longer in common use, having been replaced by more useful tests.

Iron

Small amounts of iron are carried in the serum in combination with the proteins. This iron is in balance with the iron concentration in the rest of the body, and variations in its levels can reflect disturbances in other areas of iron storage and utilization. In iron deficiency (microcytic) anemia, the serum iron levels will be lower than normal. The levels are higher than normal in hemolytic disorders, in untreated macrocytic anemias, and in hemochromatosis (a condition of excess iron deposition in the liver and elsewhere).

Food and drink restrictions   None.

Procedure for collecting specimen   Collect *venous* blood in a collecting tube with a red stopper. Most laboratories require 10 ml.

Laboratory procedure   Several procedures are available. The most commonly used procedures are colorimetric.

Possible interfering materials and conditions   A patient who has been anemic, and has recently begun to correct the anemia by more red blood cell production following the administration of cyanocobalamin (Vitamin B_{12}) or folic acid, may have low serum iron levels despite an adequate iron balance.

Hemolysis of the sample will produce a falsely elevated reading. The serum iron level may be elevated by oral contraceptives.

Normal range   *Adults:* 60 to 200 mcg/100 ml serum. *Children:* 55 to 185 mcg/100 ml serum.

Iron-Binding Capacity (Unsaturated)

This test measures the amount of extra iron that could be carried in the plasma. Iron is transported in plasma by a protein, transferrin (also called siderophilin). Ordinarily, the actual serum iron is about one-third the level of the total iron-binding capacity. The measurement of unsaturated iron-binding capacity is particularly useful in the early diagnosis of hemochromatosis, a condition in which excess iron deposited in vital tissues interferes with their function. If diagnosed early enough, suitable therapeutic measures can be most helpful. In hemochromatosis, the transferrin is highly saturated with iron, so that the unsaturated iron-binding capacity is quite low. There is also some lowering of unsaturated iron-binding capacity in pernicious anemia, hemolytic anemia, cirrhosis of the liver, uremia, and some infections. Unsaturated iron-binding capacity may be increased in iron deficiency anemia, in acute chronic blood loss, and in pregnancy.

Food and drink restrictions   None.

Procedure for collecting specimen   Collect *venous* blood in a collecting tube with a red stopper. Most laboratories require 10 ml but micromethods are also available.

Laboratory procedure   A known quantity of iron salt is added to the serum, and the amount that is not bound to transferrin is measured in a spectrophotometer.

Possible interfering materials and conditions   The iron-binding capacity may be elevated by oral contraceptives.

Hemolysis of the sample will make accurate readings impossible.

Normal range   *Adults:* 250 to 425 mcg/100 ml. *Children:* Same as the range for adults.

Kahn   *See* Serological Tests for Syphilis

Ketone Bodies

This is a test for serious metabolic abnormalities, particularly diabetic acidosis. The ketone bodies—betahydroxybutyric acid, acetoacetic (diacetic) acid, and acetone—are generally produced by fat metabolism and cause acidosis. In conditions such as severe diabetes and starvation, there is little carbohydrate to metabolize, so fats are used excessively, producing excessive ketone bodies. Ordinarily, there are only small levels of ketone bodies in the blood, less than 4 mg/100 ml or 0.4 mEq/L. In diabetic acidosis, a life-threatening situation, levels of 50 to 400 mg/100 ml or 5 to 40 mEq/L may be seen.

This test is not usually used to diagnose starvation because that condition would be obvious by the time ketonemia is present. Some hospitals test separately for acetone and acetoacetic acid.

Food and drink restrictions None.

Procedure for collecting specimen Collect 3 ml of *venous* blood in a collecting tube with a red stopper.

Laboratory procedure The ketone bodies in the sample, under heat, change a colorless compound to a colored one, and the degree of change is measured in a spectrophotometer.

Possible interfering materials and conditions None reported yet.

Normal range Expressed in milligrams per 100 milliliters (mg/100 ml) or milliequivalents per liter (mEq/L).

Adults: 2 to 4 mg/100 ml *or*
0.2 to 0.4 mEq/L

Children: Newborn to 1 week: Slightly higher than adult range
Over 1 week: Similar to adult range

Kolmer *See* Serological Tests for Syphilis

Lactic Dehydrogenase

This test is used primarily as an aid in the diagnosis of myocardial infarction. Lactic dehydrogenases are enzymes found in serum and in several organs including the heart. Therefore, an increase in levels of lactic dehydrogenase is not specific but, in conjunction with other tests, can help diagnose the presence of myocardial infarction. After an infarction occurs, the serum level of lactic dehydrogenase shows a perceptible rise in 6 to 12 hours, and may reach levels of from 2 to 10 times normal in 1 to 3 days. The elevated levels persist from 1 to 3 weeks after the infarction. There may also be markedly elevated levels in untreated acute leukemia, malignant lymphoma, megaloblastic anemia, sickle-cell anemia, liver disease, and extensive carcinomas. There is some disagreement about whether the levels are elevated in pulmonary infarction.

Food and drink restrictions None.

Procedure for collecting specimen Collect 5 ml of *venous* blood in a collecting tube with a red stopper.

Laboratory procedure Both colorimetric and spectrophotometric procedures are available.

Possible interfering materials and conditions If any oxalate comes in contact with the specimen, it will cause falsely low readings. The red blood cells contain high levels of the enzyme, and if hemolysis occurs, high levels may be obtained as an artifact.

Normal range *Adults:* At least three different types of units are used for reporting lactic dehydrogenase levels, so one must be sure which unit is referred to. Probably the most common now is the International Unit. However, there is an enormous range of values in use by different hospital laboratories even when International Units are specified. Five large hospital laboratories were compared, and only two of them used values that were similar. The normal values given went from 130 to 330 IU per liter to 15 to 60 IU per milliliter, more than a 100-fold difference. Accordingly, until there is a better standardization, one must check to find the normal range used by the particular laboratory. *Children:* Usually the same as the adult range in most laboratories.

Lactic Dehydrogenase, Heat-Stable *See* Heat-Stable Lactic Dehydrogenase

Lactic Dehydrogenase Isoenzymes (LDH Isoenzymes)

The lactic dehydrogenases can be divided into five components that are present in different concentrations in different tissues and organs. For example, the myocardium has large amounts of isoenzymes 1 and 2, but only traces of isoenzymes 4 and 5. On the other hand, the liver has large concentrations of isoenzyme 5, but only traces of isoenzymes 1 and 2. By studying the pattern of concentrations of the isoenzymes, it is possible to get much more specific diagnostic information than is provided by the regular lactic dehydrogenase measurement alone.

At this time, the measurement and comparison of all the isoenzyme concentrations is complex and difficult and, as a result, complete analysis of the isoenzymes is not commonly done. However, this procedure is becoming more common.

At this time, the measurement of isoenzyme 1, also known as "Heat-Stable Lactic Dehydrogenase," is still used (see p. 73) for diagnosing myocardial infarction. Information is rapidly being accumulated about the significance of increased levels of the other isoenzymes.

Elevated levels of isoenzyme 2 also occur in myocardial infarction. Elevated levels of isoenzyme 3 are found in pulmonary infarction. Elevated levels of isoenzyme 4 and 5 are found in liver disease and in chemical poisoning of the liver. There are other conditions in which levels of two or more isoenzymes are elevated.

Food and drink restrictions   None.

Procedure for collecting specimen   Collect at least 5 ml of *venous* blood in a collecting tube with a red stopper.

Laboratory procedure   Many laboratories use electrophoresis.

Possible interfering materials and conditions   A number of disease conditions are known to change the isoenzyme pattern, and there is a strong probability that other disease conditions will also be found to do so. Therefore, the laboratory should be informed of *all* the diseases and pathologic conditions a patient has, not merely the one of immediate concern.

Normal range   This varies from laboratory to laboratory. Representative levels (expressed as percentages) are listed below.

Adults:	Fraction 1	25 to 33
	Fraction 2	35 to 41
	Fraction 3	16 to 22
	Fraction 4	6 to 10
	Fraction 5	3 to 7

Children: This test is not usually performed on children, and normal values have not been established.

Latex Slide Agglutination   *See* Rheumatoid Arthritis Test

LD   *See* Lactic Dehydrogenase

LDH   *See* Lactic Dehydrogenase

LE   *See* Lupus Erythematosus Cell Test

Lead

The usual use for this test is in suspected cases of acute lead poisoning, or an acute episode superimposed on chronic lead intoxication. This is a particularly important test in some areas of rundown housing in which children may eat peeling lead-based paint.

Food and drink restrictions   None.

Procedure for collecting specimen   Collect *venous* blood in a collecting tube with a green or brown stopper (check with the laboratory). The tube should be filled. In some hospital laboratories micromethods are available.

Laboratory procedure   Both chemical and spectrographic methods are available.

Possible interfering materials and conditions   None reported.

Normal range   Expressed in milligrams *or* micrograms per 100 milliliters of whole blood.

Adults: 0 to 0.08 mg/100 ml
0 to 80 mcg/100 ml
Some hospitals consider 40 mcg/100 ml to be the upper limit of normal.

Children: Same as that for adults.

Leucine Aminopeptidase

This test is no longer in use.

Leukocyte Count   *See* Blood Counts, White Cell Count

Lipase

This is a test for damage to the pancreas. Like amylase, lipase is secreted by the pancreas, and small amounts pass into the blood. In diseases such as acute pancreatitis and carcinoma of the pancreas, the blood level of lipase rises. Both amylase and lipase levels rise at the same rate, but the elevation in lipase concentration persists for a longer period. Therefore, the lipase determination is made when too much time has elapsed for the amylase level to remain elevated.

Food and drink restrictions It is not clear whether or not the eating of food interferes with this test, since the test itself is not considered precise or completely accurate. It would probably be best, when practical, to draw the serum sample before breakfast after an overnight fast. If this cannot be done, a note should be made in the chart, indicating when the sample was drawn in relation to the last meal. Water may be taken freely.

Procedure for collecting specimen Collect *venous* blood in a collecting tube with a red stopper. Various laboratories require different amounts. The largest amount required by any laboratory is 10 ml.

Laboratory procedure The serum sample is incubated with an oil. The amount of fatty acid liberated is titrated.

Possible interfering materials and conditions Serum lipase levels may be elevated into a distinctly abnormal range if the patient has received bethanechol (Myocholine, Urecholine), codeine, or morphine. Although definite evidence is not available, it seems prudent to assume that the other narcotic drugs may also produce falsely high levels of serum lipase if taken within the 24 hours before the sample is drawn.

Normal range *Adults:* Not over 1.5 units/ml. *Children:* This test is not ordinarily performed on children and normal values have not been definitely established.

Lipid Fractions

This test measures the amounts of the several lipid fractions in the serum. Lipids are substances that are chemically related to fatty acids. In certain diseases, one or more lipid fraction concentrations are elevated. For example, in hypothyroidism, cholesterol is elevated; in nephrotic syndrome, total lipids are extremely high; in glycogen storage diseases and in ketosis, total lipids are elevated. There are, in addition, at least 5 primary, congenital types of hyperlipemia in which the lipids are carried bound to protein (hyperlipoproteinemias) that require additional tests for diagnosis. There is also substantial evidence that atherosclerosis is related to excess concentration of one or more lipid fractions in the serum, but the precise relationship is still unproven. Often a physician orders a measurement of lipid fractions in the hope that it will furnish a clue to the management of a patient with actual or suspected atherosclerosis.

Food and drink restrictions   The patient should be on a normal diet for 3 weeks before the test, and must fast for 12 hours before the blood sample is drawn. Water may be taken ad lib.

Procedure for collecting specimen   Collect 10 ml of *venous* blood in a collecting tube with a red stopper.

Laboratory procedure   Each lipid fraction is measured by a different chemical procedure, all of them quite complex.

Possible interfering materials and conditions   None reported yet.

Normal range   There is considerable variation among laboratories. The ranges given below (in milligrams per 100 milliliters and milliequivalents per liter) encompass most, but not all, laboratories. Normal values for the laboratory reporting should be determined.

Adults:	total lipids	400 to 800 mg/100 ml
	phospholipids	150 to 380 mg/100 ml
	cholesterol, total	120 to 260 mg/100 ml
		(*see also* Cholesterol, p. 54)
	cholesterol, free	up to 50 mg/100 ml
	cholesterol, esters	up to 210 mg/100 ml
	triglycerides (neutral fat)	25 to 150 mg/100 ml
	free fatty acids	0.3 to 1.0 mEq/L

Children: Similar to the range for adults, except for cholesterol (see p. 54).

Lipoprotein Analysis

This is a test to determine the presence or absence of certain disorders of fat metabolism. The lipids, which include fats and related compounds, are generally found in combination with one or more of the serum proteins. The combination of lipid and protein is called lipoprotein. At least 5 different types of familial disorder of lipid and lipoprotein metabolism are known. They are designated as I, II, III, IV, and V. Prognosis and management differ for each, and it is therefore helpful to know exactly which type of disorder a particular patient has. In addition, there may be other types of either familial or acquired lipoprotein disorder that have not yet been classified.

Food and drink restrictions   The patient should be on a normal diet for 3 weeks before the test, and must fast for 12 hours before the blood sample is drawn. Water may be taken ad lib.

Procedure for collecting specimen   Collect *venous* blood in a collecting tube with a red stopper. Most laboratories need 4 ml, but some require more.

Laboratory procedure   The sample is subjected to electrophoresis, and the lipoprotein bands compared to standards.

Possible interfering materials and conditions   None reported yet.

Normal range   The normal range is determined by comparison with standard electrophoresis patterns.

Lithium

This test is used to monitor the lithium dosage in treatment of manic-depressive psychosis. Lithium, the lightest metal, forms salts that are similar to sodium salts. Once used as a sodium substitute in some diets, lithium salts were abandoned in the 1940s because their toxicity was too high when compared to the benefits. Then, in 1949, Dr. Cade in Australia found that lithium salts can correct the mania in manic depression, and it was also discovered that lithium can help prevent the depression. The seriousness of manic-depression is so great that the toxicity of lithium salts is not a contraindication to their use in this condition.

Ironically, because of poor coordination and information exchange among scientists, Cade's great discovery was ignored in this country for more than 15 years, and only now are patients deriving benefit from it. The serum concentration of lithium must be kept within rather close limits to be effective and yet nontoxic. Therefore, patients receiving lithium salts must have serum levels checked regularly. The therapeutic level ranges from 0.6 to 1.6 mEq/L. At levels over 2.0 mEq/L, severe toxicity may occur, and dosage must be stopped or reduced.

Food and drink restrictions   None reported, but there are restrictions on intake of medication.

Procedure for collecting specimen   The patient must not have taken any lithium in the preceding 8 hours. Collect 5 ml of *venous* blood in a collecting tube with a red stopper.

Laboratory procedure   The serum concentration of lithium is measured in a flame photometer.

Possible interfering materials and conditions   None reported yet.

Normal range   *Adults:* Normally, there is no measurable lithium in the serum. The *therapeutic* levels in patients are 0.5 to 1.5 mEq/L. (Some physicians try for a level of 0.5 to 1.0 mEq/L. *Children:* Lithium is not ordinarily given to children.

Lupus Erythematosus (LE) Cell Test

A particular type of cell called the lupus erythematosus cell is often seen in lupus erythematosus. Finding this cell can help in the diagnosis, although it may also be found in other conditions.

Food and drink restrictions   None.

Procedure for collecting specimen   Some laboratories use clotted and others use unclotted blood. The color of the stopper of the collecting tube to be used varies with different laboratories.

Laboratory procedure   The leucocytes of the blood are concentrated by centrifugation, smeared, and stained. The stained smears are then examined microscopically for LE cells.

Possible interfering materials and conditions   None reported yet.

Normal range   *Adults:* Normally there are no lupus erythematosus cells in the blood. *Children:* Same as for adults.

Magnesium

In magnesium deficiency, a state of tetany can sometimes occur, which in appearance is indistinguishable from the tetany of low calcium. Accordingly, in tetanic or pretetanic conditions, serum magnesium levels may be measured to see whether they are abnormally low. If they are, magnesium salts usually correct the symptoms. In patients receiving large amounts of parenteral fluids for long periods, serum magnesium levels may be measured in an attempt to diagnose an early magnesium deficiency and correct it before tetany occurs.

Food and drink restrictions   None.

Procedure for collecting specimen   Collect 3 ml of *venous* blood in a collecting tube with a red stopper.

Laboratory procedure   There are several methods available for determination of magnesium levels. Atomic absorption spectrophotometry is the method of choice.

Possible interfering materials and conditions   None reported yet.

Normal range   Expressed in milligrams per 100 milliliters of serum, *or* milliequivalents per liter of serum.

Adults: 1.8 to 3.0 mg/100 ml *or*
         1.5 to 2.5 mEq/L

Children: 2.0 to 2.6 mg/100 ml *or*
         1.7 to 2.2 mEq/L

Malaria Film

This is a test for malarial parasites in the blood. It is important not only in establishing a definite diagnosis of malaria but also in determining which species of malarial parasite is involved. Each species can be identified on the film.

Food and drink restrictions   None.

Procedure for collecting specimen   Collect *venous* blood in a collecting tube with a lavender stopper. The tube should be at least half full.

Laboratory procedure   A film of blood is placed on a slide, stained, and examined microscopically. If the first smears are negative, they may be repeated 6 to 12 hours after a chill, when there is a greater likelihood of finding the parasites in the blood.

Possible interfering materials and conditions   None reported yet.

Normal range   Normally there are no malarial parasites in the blood.

Mazzini   *See* Serological Tests for Syphilis

Methemoglobin

Methemoglobin is not ordinarily present in the blood. It is found when the hemoglobin is oxidized by chemicals such as nitrites, chlorates, etc. Drinking well water containing nitrites is a frequent cause of methemoglobinemia. Methemoglobin is not an oxygen carrier as is hemoglobin.

Food and drink restrictions   None.

Procedure for collecting specimen   Collect *venous* blood in a collecting tube with a green or lavender stopper, depending on the laboratory. The tube should be filled.

Laboratory procedure   Methemoglobin is detected by the use of the spectroscope.

Possible interfering materials and conditions   None reported yet.

Normal range   Normally there is no methemoglobin in the blood.

Mono-Diff

This is a commercially available test for infectious mononucleosis. It is performed on a slide, using a few drops of blood, and can be read in two minutes. It is, therefore, suitable for physicians' offices and clinics.

Food and drink restrictions   None.

Procedure for collecting specimen   Collect 2 ml of *venous* blood in a collecting tube with a red stopper.

Laboratory procedure   This is described in steps by the manufacturer of the equipment used in making the test.

Possible interfering materials and conditions None reported yet.

Normal range *Adults* and *Children:* Negative.

Nonprotein Nitrogen (NPN)

This test is similar to, but less accurate and less specific than, the blood urea nitrogen (BUN) test. Accordingly, it is no longer in common use.

NPN *See* Nonprotein Nitrogen

OGTT *See* Glucose Tolerance

Osmolality, Serum

The term ''osmolality'' is related to, but slightly different from, ''osmolarity.'' A ''molar'' solution contains a mol (or osmol) of dissolved material in one liter of *solution*. A ''molal'' solution contains a mol (or osmol) of dissolved material in one kilogram of *solvent*. Although these distinctions are important in physical chemistry, they are of no practical significance in clinical evaluation. A value for serum expressed in *molar* terms would only differ by 1 milliosmol from the value expressed in *molal* terms.

The osmolality of serum indicates in a general way the amount of material dissolved in the serum. However, because of physicochemical laws, the osmolality does not always have a simple linear relation to the amount of solute. For example, if the osmolality of one solution is twice the osmolality of another solution, that doesn't mean that the first solution has twice the solutes of the other solution. This is true even if the solutes in the two solutions are identical and are present in identical proportions.

A knowledge of the serum osmolality is helpful in the diagnosis of electrolyte and fluid disorders. A decreased serum osmolality is caused by low sodium concentrations. An increased serum osmolality may be seen in dehydration, sodium overload, hyperglycemia, uremia, and some other conditions.

Food and drink restrictions None.

Procedure for collecting specimen   Collect *venous* blood in a collecting tube with a red stopper. Five to ten ml are needed, depending on the laboratory.

Laboratory procedure   A common method is the determination of the freezing point of the sample. Vapor pressure measurements may become the method of the future.

Possible interfering materials and conditions   None reported yet.

Normal range   *Adults:* 275-295 milliosmols/kg water. *Children:* 270-285 milliosmols/kg water.

Partial Thromboplastin Time (PTT)

This is a sophisticated test for certain defects in the coagulation system. Thromboplastin is that part of tissue and/or platelet extracts that accelerates the clotting process. The term "complete thromboplastin" refers to a tissue extract that can clot plasma from hemophiliac patients as rapidly as plasma from normal persons. The term "partial thromboplastin" refers to an extract (usually from platelets) that clots hemophiliac plasma at a slower rate than normal plasma. The partial thromboplastin time test may be used by itself as a screening test to pick up a coagulation defect. However, mild coagulation defects may be missed.

In the classification of some of the more complex bleeding conditions, the activated partial thromboplastin time, in conjunction with results of the prothrombin time test and other related tests, can usually suggest the diagnosis. Deficiencies in Factors I, II, V, VII, VIII, IX, or X can usually be spotted, depending on the combination of results of the various tests. No one test, however, can indicate the correct diagnosis, and the interpretation of the meaning of the pattern in test results usually requires an experienced hematologist.

Food and drink restrictions   None.

Procedure for collecting specimen   Collect *venous* blood in the same test tube used for collecting a specimen for prothrombin time; it should have a blue stopper. A special oxalate solution is used as an anticoagulant. The tube must be filled to capacity.

Laboratory procedure   To a measured sample of the patient's plasma, measured amounts of calcium chloride and partial thromboplastin suspension are added in a predetermined sequence. The time that elapses until formation of a fibrin clot is measured by a stop-watch.

Possible interfering materials and conditions   None reported yet.

Normal range   *Adults:* The results must be compared with those obtained the same day, in the same laboratory, with normal human plasma. There are differences from hospital to hospital, depending on the preparation of thromboplastin used.

Normally, adult human plasma has a PTT of under 38 seconds. Anything over 44 seconds is considered abnormal in some laboratories. In others, the limit of normality is 46. *Children:* Similar to that of adults.

Paul-Bunnell Test   *See* Heterophile Antibody

PBI   *See* Protein-Bound Iodine

Partial Pressure of Carbon Dioxide (PCO₂)

This is a measure of the partial pressure of carbon dioxide in a gas phase in equilibrium with blood. It is usually measured on arterial blood, although deep capillary blood is sometimes used. Levels of arterial PCO_2 above normal may stem from a congenital cardiovascular defect, interference with respiratory exchange, or various lung disorders. Interpretation of the significance of abnormal PCO_2 levels, therefore, depends on correlation with clinical findings and with the PO_2 (partial pressure of oxygen) and pH. The physician may designate this test "emergency."

Food and drink restrictions   None reported.

Procedure for collecting specimen   The patient should be at rest for at least 15 minutes. The sample of *arterial* blood is collected by a physician, preferably in a heparinized vacutainer tube. Many hospital laboratories use a collecting tube with green stopper. The tube should be completely filled with blood and iced. In some laboratories, a heparinized syringe is used.

Laboratory procedure   The PCO_2 is measured directly on an electronic meter consisting of a pH meter adapted for PCO_2 measurements.

Possible interfering materials and conditions　None reported.

Normal range　*Adults:* Normally, the *arterial* PCO_2 is 35-40 mm Hg. *Children:* Normally the *arterial* PCO_2 is 35 to 43 mm Hg.

PCV (Packed Cell Volume)　*See* Hematocrit

pH

This is a measure of acidity or alkalinity. The normal blood pH ranges from 7.35 to 7.45. The pH may be lower in such conditions as hypoventilation, severe diarrhea, Addison's disease, and diabetic acidosis. The pH may rise above normal levels in conditions such as excess vomiting, Cushing's syndrome, and hyperventilation.

Food and drink restrictions　None.

Procedure for collecting specimen　Collect 5 ml of *venous* blood in a collecting tube with a green stopper. The blood should be withdrawn without using a tourniquet, if possible. If a tourniquet is necessary, the patient should *not* open and close his fist, but should keep it closed without straining.

Laboratory procedure　A sensitive pH meter measures the pH electronically.

Possible interfering materials and conditions　None reported yet.

Normal range　*Adults:* pH 7.35 to 7.45. *Children:* pH 7.38 to 7.42.

Phenylketonuria　*See* Guthrie

Phosphatase, Acid

This is a test to identify metastasizing carcinomas of the prostate. Normally, small amounts of acid phosphatase are found in the serum. The prostate gland is exceptionally rich in this enzyme and so are carcinomas of the prostate. The normal gland and the carcinoma that has not yet spread do not release the enzyme into the serum. However, the metastasizing prostate carcinoma does, thereby increasing the serum concentration markedly. The test is performed only on men. Besides carcinoma of the prostate, other conditions that produce elevated serum acid phosphatase levels include: Paget's disease, hyperparathyroidism, metastatic mammary carcinoma, multiple myeloma, some liver diseases, renal insufficiency, osteogenesis imperfecta, thrombocytosis, arterial embolism, myocardial infarction, thrombophlebitis, pulmonary embolism, and sickle-cell crisis.

Food and drink restrictions   None.

Procedure for collecting specimen   Collect 5 ml of *venous* blood in a collecting tube with a red stopper.

Laboratory procedure   The speed with which a sample of serum hydrolyzes a monophosphate ester at pH 5 is measured.

Possible interfering materials and conditions   If the patient has had a prostatic massage, or extensive palpation of the prostate, there may be elevation of the serum acid phosphatase to abnormal levels for about 24 hours.

Hemolysis of the specimen can produce spuriously high levels.

Clofibrate (atromid-S) may give a spuriously high level of acid phosphatase.

The following may give a spurious decrease of acid phophatase levels: fluorides, oxalates, phosphates.

Normal range   Some laboratories use International Units, but from laboratory to laboratory, the normal ranges vary by more than an order of magnitude. Therefore, there appears to be some ambiguity about the meaning of International Unit in this test and, if the laboratory uses an International Unit, one must determine what the laboratory's normal range is. Furthermore, one must not assume that an International Unit in one laboratory means the same as an International Unit in another laboratory as far as this test is concerned.

Adults: up to 4 King-Armstrong units/ml *or*
up to 1.1 Bodansky units/ml *or*
up to .63 Bessey-Lowry units/ml

Children: This test is not usually performed on children.

Phosphatase, Alkaline

This test may be used in the diagnosis of bone as well as of liver diseases. Normally, there is a small amount of alkaline phosphatase in the serum. In bone diseases, however, the alkaline phosphatase rises in proportion to the formation of new bone cells. This test, therefore, may be of value in differentiating between various bone disorders, including tumors. In disorders of the liver and biliary tract, the alkaline phosphatase rises because excretion is impaired. This test may therefore also be of some use in evaluating the degree of blockage of the biliary tract.

The alkaline phosphatase levels are elevated in hyperparathyroidism, osteitis deformans, osteomalacia, Gaucher's disease, rickets, healing fractures, Boeck's sarcoid, hyperthyroidism (Grave's disease), leukemia, after administration of large amounts of vitamin D, and in pregnancy.

Food and drink restrictions   None.

Procedure for collecting specimen   Collect 5 ml of *venous* blood in a collecting tube with a red stopper.

Laboratory procedure   The speed with which a sample of serum hydrolyzes a phosphate ester at pH 9.7 is measured.

Possible interfering materials and conditions   The alkaline phosphatase levels may be elevated by several drugs. In some cases, the elevation results from an action of the drug on body enzymes, but the increased level does not indicate bone or liver disease. Because the number of drugs that cause elevation of alkaline phosphatase levels is large, only official (generic) names are listed:

acetohexamide	methyldopa
allopurinol	n-hydroxyacetamide
anabolic agents (some)	oral contraceptives (some)
androgens, some	oxacillin
chlorpropamide	penicillamine
colchicine	phenothiazines (some)
erythromycin	procainamide
gold salts	thiothixene
indomethacin	tolazamide
lincomycin	tolbutamide

Large amounts of vitamin D can also produce elevations in the serum level of alkaline phosphatase.

Normal range   Some laboratories use units other than those listed below, including International Units. As is the case with the Acid Phosphatase test, there is no agreement on the size of these units, and the variation from laboratory to laboratory is extremely wide. Therefore, one must find out the normal range for the laboratory providing the test. Furthermore, one cannot assume that a unit has the same meaning in two laboratories, even if both are called International Units.

Adults: King-Armstrong units   4 to 13/100 ml *or*
Bodansky units   1.5 to 4.5/100 ml *or*
Bessy-Lowry units   0.8 to 2.3/ml

Children: The normal range in children is generally much higher than in adults because of rapid bone growth in children. In many, the highest level is found at ages 11 to 14, but bone growth rather than chronological age is the major factor. The normal ranges are:

King-Armstrong units   15 to 30/100 ml *or*
Bodansky units   5 to 14/100 ml *or*
Bessy-Lowry units   3 to 9/ml

Phosphorus (Inorganic)

Phosphorus metabolism is directly associated with calcium metabolism and involves many organs and physiological functions. The concentration of phosphorus may be increased in severe kidney disease, hypoparathyroidism, acromegaly, or excessive vitamin D intake. The concentration may decrease in rickets, hyperparathyroidism, and certain diseases of the kidney tubules.

Food and drink restrictions It is best to draw the blood sample in the morning after an overnight fast, but not all laboratories require this.

Procedure for collecting specimen Collect 5 ml of *venous* blood in a collecting tube with a red stopper. Hemolysis must be avoided.

Laboratory procedure A colorimetric method is usually used, but there are several variations among laboratories.

Possible interfering materials and conditions The phophorus level may be elevated if the patient has recently received diphenylhydantoin (Dilantin), heparin, pituitrin, or vitamin D. It may be interfered with or increased if the patient has recently received

epinephrine (Adrenalin) or insulin. Hemolysis may produce spuriously high levels.

Normal range   Expressed in milliequivalents per liter *or* milligrams per 100 milliliters.

Adults: 1.8 to 2.6 mEq/L *or*
            3.0 to 4.5 mg/100 ml

Children: Newborn: 2.4 to 5.9 mEq/L *or*
                         4 to 10 mg/100 ml

              Others: 2.4 to 4.1 mEq/L *or*
                         4 to 7 mg/100 ml

Platelet Count   *See* Blood Counts, Platelet Count

Plasma Electrophoresis for Gammopathies   *See* Immunoglobulins

PO$_2$

This is a measure of the partial pressure of oxygen in the gas phase in
equilibrium with blood. It is usually measured on arterial blood,
although deep capillary blood is sometimes used. Levels of PO$_2$
below normal may stem from a variety of conditions such as congenital heart defects, interference with respiratory exchange, and a variety of lung disorders. Interpretation of the significance of abnormal
PO$_2$ levels therefore depends on correlation with clinical findings
and with the PCO$_2$ and pH. The physician may designate this test
"emergency."

Food and drink restrictions   None reported.

Procedure for collecting specimen   The patient should be at rest
for at least 15 minutes before the physician collects the sample of
arterial blood in a collecting tube with a green stopper. The tube
should be filled completely and placed in ice at once.

Laboratory procedure   The PO$_2$ is measured directly on an electronic meter consisting of a pH meter adapted for PO$_2$ measurements.

Possible interfering materials and conditions   None reported
yet.

Normal range   *Adults:* There appear to be substantial variations between laboratories. A standard text gives a normal range of 75 to 100 mm Hg. However, some laboratories use 80 to 90 mm Hg, and other 90 to 110 mm Hg, as the normal range. *Children:* The normal range should be similar for children, but it varies from laboratory to laboratory.

Potassium

Potassium is an essential ion found in large concentrations in all cells and in much smaller concentrations in the serum. Alterations in serum potassium levels may produce serious changes in body function, or even death. A marked decrease in serum potassium may cause cardiac arrhythmias and muscle weakness; a marked increase produces a series of electrocardiographic changes and arrhythmias. There may also be depression, lethargy, and coma. Therefore, when it is suspected that serum potassium levels have changed, tests should be made and measures taken to restore them to the normal range. Increased serum potassium levels may be found in conditions of severe cell damage and destruction, adrenal cortical deficiency, and hypoventilation. A decrease in serum potassium may be found in severe diarrhea, periodic familial paralysis, chronic kidney disease, excess function of the adrenal cortex, and following administration of insulin and glucose in diabetes without added potassium. Low serum potassium levels are particularly dangerous when digitalis glycosides are being administered.

It has been reported that low serum potassium levels in the presence of hypertension suggest primary aldosteronism.

Food and drink restrictions   None.

Procedure for collecting specimen   Collect 5 ml of *venous* blood in a collecting tube with a red stopper.

Laboratory procedure   The serum concentration of potassium is measured in a flame photometer.

Possible interfering materials and conditions   The serum potassium level may be elevated by tobacco smoke. It may be decreased by several drugs. However, this decrease is a true decrease in the actual potassium level, and not a spurious or misleading effect on a test procedure. The fact that these drugs have such effects cannot be considered as interference with test results; indeed, many times the test is ordered by the doctor precisely because he wishes to know the extent to which a prescribed drug is affecting serum potassium levels. The materials having such an effect include acetazolamide, ACTH, cortisone and some of its derivatives, P-aminosalicylic acid, and glucose.

Normal range   *Adults:* A common normal range is 3.8 to 5 mEq/L. However, some laboratories consider as normal a range as wide as 3.6 to 5.5 mEq/L. *Children:* Approximately the same as the range for adults.

Protein-Bound Iodine (PBI)

This test of thyroid function is being replaced by more exact tests. However, it is still used in some laboratories.

The thyroid gland binds iodine to organic compounds, mainly to the hormone thyroxin. This hormone is precipitated by chemicals that precipitate proteins, so that a measurement of the amount of iodine in a protein precipitate indicates the amount of thyroid hormone present. An increased concentration of protein-bound iodine is usually found in hyperthyroidism, although it may also be seen in early hepatitis. A decreased concentration of protein-bound iodine is usually found in hypothyroidism.

Food and drink restrictions   None.

Procedure for collecting specimen   The patient must not have received any iodine-containing drugs or any iodine-containing contrast media for the appropriate period before performing this test (see Table 22). Collect 8 ml of *venous* blood in a collecting tube with a red stopper.

Laboratory procedure   A protein precipitant is added to a sample of serum and the precipitate removed, washed, treated with alkali, and redissolved. Its ability to decolorize a yellow solution of ceric sulfate indicates the iodine content.

Possible interfering materials and conditions   The protein-bound iodine levels are affected by so many medications that special efforts should be made to see that the patient does not take medications or receive radiographic contrast media for several days before the test. Unfortunately, some radiographic contrast media can produce false high results for long periods. In general, it should be assumed that all radiopaque, iodine-containing injectable contrast media are likely to produce falsely elevated protein-bound iodine levels for 6 months. Some of these contrast media are believed to exert an effect for 20 or more years. The number of drugs affecting protein-bound iodine levels is so extensive that a listing of many of the brand names is not feasible. Accordingly, only official names will be presented.

The drugs and foods which can produce a misleading *elevation* of the protein bound-iodine include:

barbiturates (see Table 18)
barium sulfate (use in GI
   series and barium enema)
estrogens (see Table 21)
gargles, some
iodine-containing drugs
   (see Table 22)
lithium carbonate capsule
   dye
Metrecal
mouth washes, some
oral contraceptives
perphenazine
sun-tan lotions, some

The protein-bound iodine may be spuriously elevated if a patient has had intravenous solutions given by catheter before the sample is drawn. Iodine is leached out of the catheter in amounts sufficient to alter test results.

In biliary tract obstruction, there may be a spurious elevation of the protein-bound iodine.

The drugs that can produce misleading *depression* of protein-bound iodine levels include:

ACTH
androgens (see Table 16)
cortisone-like drugs (see
   Table 20)
diphenylhydantoin
disulfiram
gold salts (for weeks or
   months)
isoniazid
liothyronine
mercurial diuretics
para-aminobenzoic acid
para-aminosalicylic acid
phenothiazines except
   perphenazine
phenylbutazone
reserpine
salicylates, including aspirin
   (see Table 27)
sulfonamides
thiazides
thiocyanates
tri-iodothyronine
vitamin preparations, some

In addition, the Bromsulphalein retention test (BSP) may produce false elevations or depressions of the protein-bound iodine levels.

Normal range   *Adults:* 4 to 8 mcg/100 ml serum. *Children:* Similar to that for adults.

Protein, Total   *See* Albumin, Globulin, Total Protein, A/G Ratio

Prothrombin Time

This is an indirect test of the clotting ability of the blood. Prothrombin is converted to thrombin in the clotting process. When the prothrombin level of the blood is lower than normal, it is believed that the clotting tendency of the blood within the blood vessels is diminished. The prothrombin content of the blood is lowered in liver diseases, hypoprothrombinemia of infants, vitamin K deficiency, and following drug therapy. The vast majority of cases of low blood prothrombin results from the administration of Dicumarol or similar drugs. The substances are given to reduce the clotting tendency of the blood and thus avoid thromboembolic phenomena.

This test is often done daily during the acute stages of myocardial infarction, and accurate results are needed promptly in order to enable the physician to determine the size of the next dose of anticoagulant.

Food and drink restrictions   None.

Procedure for collecting specimen   Collect *venous* blood in a collecting tube with a blue stopper. The tube must be filled to capacity.

Laboratory procedure   Of several available methods, the most commonly used is the one-stage method of Quick, in which a mixture of thromboplastin and calcium is added to the oxalated serum. The time that elapses until the formation of fibrin threads is measured with a stop-watch. This result is then compared to that obtained on normal blood.

Possible interfering materials and conditions   The prothrombin time may be falsely elevated by barbiturates (see Table 18).

If the vacuum tube used to collect the specimen is not completely filled, the prothrombin time may be spuriously elevated because of the effect of extra anticoagulant in the tube.

The prothrombin time may be reduced by several groups of drugs, but it is not yet clear whether the reduction is an interference with a laboratory test or whether it represents a true reduction in prothrombin levels via a biochemical effect on physiologic functions, or on indigenous bacteria. Drugs that may reduce the prothrombin time include:

> antibiotics
> hydroxyzine (Vistaril)
> salicylates, including aspirin
>   (see Table 27)
> sulfonamides

Normal range   *Adults:* Between 11 and 18 seconds, depending on the type of thromboplastin used, is considered 100% of normal. In Dicumarol treatment, the physician tries to keep the prothrombin time at 2 to 2½ times normal. Expressed as prothrombin percentage, which is not a straight-line function of prothrombin time, a range of from 20% to 30% is sought. *Children:* This test is not usually performed on children. However, when it is, the results are compared to a normal control, performed at the same time. The normal range is then considered to be 70% to 100% of the normal control.

Rapid Plasma Reagin

This screening serologic test for syphilis is rapidly and easily carried out. However, it is not as specific as other tests and, if positive, must be confirmed by a more exact test, such as VDRL.

Food and drink restrictions   None.

Procedure for collecting specimen   Collect 5 ml of *venous* blood in a collecting tube with a red stopper.

Laboratory procedure   Commercially available kits are used.

Possible interfering materials and conditions   Not known yet.

Normal range   *Adults:* Negative. *Children:* Negative.

Red Cell Count   *See* Blood Counts, Red Cell Count

Red Cell Fragility

This test is being performed less commonly since experience has shown that it is helpful in relatively few cases. It is a test of the ability of the red blood cells to resist hemolysis in a hypotonic solution. As the concentration of salts outside the cell decreases, more water continues to pass into the cell by osmosis, and the membrane finally bursts. The salt concentration at which hemolysis occurs is taken as a measure of red blood cell fragility. Fragility is increased in congenital hemolytic jaundice and aplastic anemia.

Food and drink restrictions   None.

Procedure for collecting specimen   Collect *venous* blood in a collecting tube with a lavender stopper. The tube should be filled.

Laboratory procedure   Samples of the blood are added to solutions of sodium chloride that vary in concentration from 0.28% to 0.6%, by steps of 0.02%. After gentle mixing, the mixtures are allowed to stand for several hours. The presence of hemolysis is shown by a clear red coloration of the supernatant plasma.

Possible interfering materials and conditions   None reported yet.

Normal range   *Adults:* Slight hemolysis between 0.40% and 0.46% sodium chloride; complete hemolysis between 0.30% and 0.36% sodium chloride. *Children:* Similar to the range for adults.

Reticulocyte Count   *See* Blood Counts, Reticulocyte Count

Rh Factor   *See* Blood Types, Rh Factor

Rheumatoid Arthritis (RA) Test

In many cases of rheumatoid arthritis, the patient's serum develops antibodies that agglutinate several types of particles, ranging from bacteria to red blood cells of several species, to latex particles coated with human globulin. These antibodies are now believed to be a mixture of IgM molecules.

The exact relation of the antibodies to rheumatoid arthritis is unknown, but it has been found empirically, that the two are associated. The percentage of rheumatoid arthritis patients demonstrating a positive RA test varies from 50% to 95% depending on the stage of the disease. Early, mild cases are less likely to have a positive test.

The test is also positive in some cases of lupus erythematosus, dermatomyositis, and chronic infections. Approximately 2 to 10% of normal persons also may have a positive test. Accordingly, the rheumatoid arthritis test is suggestive only.

Food and drink restrictions   None.

Procedure for collecting specimen   Collect 5 ml of *venous* blood in a collecting tube with a red stopper.

Laboratory procedure   Several procedures are available, including the use of sensitized sheep red cells and latex particles. Card and slide tests are also available.

Possible interfering materials and conditions   Diseases such as lupus erythematosus, dermatomyositis, and chronic infections may give positive reactions.

Normal range   *Adults:* This varies considerably from laboratory to laboratory, depending on the test procedure used. *Children:* This test is not commonly done on children.

Rubella Antibody

Rubella (German measles) is usually a mild disease, but when it strikes a woman in early pregnancy, it can, and often does, produce serious deformities and functional abnormalities in the unborn child. A woman who is not immune to rubella should be immunized before she becomes pregnant. Many states now require a rubella antibody determination as well as a serologic test in women before a marriage license is issued.

The rubella virus provokes the formation of several types of antibody, and we do not yet know which type gives true protection to the fetus. Because of technical feasibility, the most widely used test measures the level of hemagglutinating antibodies. Titers of 1:64 or higher indicate definite resistance to infection. Titers below 1:8 mean susceptibility to infection. Titers between 1:8 and 1:64 are considered borderline. Women with titers between 1:8 and 1:64 cannot always be considered to be free from risk of contracting rubella when they are pregnant.

The rubella antibody titer is also measured to learn whether a woman has recently had rubella, in order to assess the need for therapeutic abortion. In general, a 4X rise in titer is considered by some authorities to mean a recent infection. Other authorities, however, do not consider a 4X rise in titer as evidence of viremia and of risk to the fetus if the patient has a history of having had rubella or has been successfully inoculated against it. This matter has not yet been resolved.

Food and drink restrictions None.

Procedure for collecting specimen Collect 3 ml of *venous* blood in a collecting tube with a red stopper.

Laboratory procedure The most common procedure is the hemagglutination-inhibition test.

Possible interfering materials and conditions None reported yet.

Normal range This depends on whether or not there has been exposure to rubella or to rubella vaccine. Experts disagree on the exact antibody titer that signifies protection of the fetus.

Salicylates

Salicylate levels may be measured in two distinct types of situations. In some cases of rheumatic fever, large doses of salicylates are used to control symptoms. The blood level of the drug may be measured in an attempt to adjust dosage more effectively. It is generally considered necessary to have blood levels of at least 25 mg/100 ml for full therapeutic effect. Unfortunately, this level may be toxic to some children.

In cases of accidental poisoning, blood salicylate levels may be helpful in making correct decisions as to management. Salicylates (primarily aspirin) are the main causes of poisoning in children. In most cases, blood levels over 35 mg/100 ml are toxic.

Food and drink restrictions None.

Procedure for collecting specimen Collect 5 ml of *venous* blood in a collecting tube with a green stopper.

Laboratory procedure Both colorimetric and spectrophotometric methods are available.

Possible interfering materials and conditions None reported yet.

Normal range *Adults:* Normally, there is no salicylate in the blood. *Children:* Same as the range for adults.

Sedimentation Rate

This test measures the rate at which red cells settle to the bottom of a glass test tube. The sedimentation rate is increased in infections and in conditions in which cell destruction occurs. This test is useful in diagnosing and following the course of such illnesses as rheumatic fever, arthritis, and myocardial infarction.

Food and drink restrictions None.

Procedure for collecting specimen Collect *venous* blood in a collecting tube with a lavender stopper. At least 4 ml are needed, and the tube should be from half full to completely full.

Laboratory procedure A sample of the blood is placed in a special thin glass tube that is kept exactly perpendicular. The rate at which the upper part of the red cell column descends is measured and is usually reported as millimeters fall in 1 hour. Corrections for anemia are sometimes made and reported as ''corrected'' sedimentation rate.

Possible interfering materials and conditions None reported yet.

Normal range *Adults:* This depends to some extent on the type of glass tube used. In the Westergren method, which is common, the normal values for men are 0 to 15 mm/hour and for women 0 to 20 mm/hour. *Children:* 0 to 20 mm/hour. A microsedimentation rate is sometimes performed. For children under 2 years, the normal range for the microsedimentation rate is 1 to 6 mm, and for those over 2 years it is 1 to 9 mm.

Serological Tests (General)

These tests are used to identify substances in the serum that result from exposure to certain microorganisms. Often, the substance to be identified and quantitated is an antibody to the microorganism itself. An example is the Widal test for typhoid antibodies. Sometimes, the material of interest is an antibody to some enzyme elaborated by a microorganism, for example, antistreptolysin O. In many cases, however, the exact relationship between the microorganism and the serological material is unknown. Years of observation have shown that, in the presence of a particular disease, the body elaborates a substance that is readily measured. For example, in infectious mononucleosis, the body produces larger amounts than usual of antibodies to sheep red blood cells (*see* Heterophile Antibody). Similarly, we do not understand the relationship of the serological tests for syphilis to the Treponema that causes the disease.

Food and drink restrictions   None.

Procedure for collecting specimen   Collect 5 ml of *venous* blood in a collecting tube with a red stopper.

Laboratory procedure   This varies with the type of test.

Possible interfering materials and conditions   None reported yet.

Normal range   There may be weak positive reactions to some serological tests in the absence of disease.

Serological Tests for Syphilis

There are several varieties, including the Wassermann, Kolmer, Kahn, Hinton, Rapid Plasma Reagin, Mazzini, and VDRL (Venereal Disease Research Laboratory) tests. All are nonspecific in nature and sometimes they are positive in diseases other than syphilis. Interpretation of these serological tests usually requires considerable skill and experience, as well as correlation with the clinical findings and history. In early primary syphilis the serology is negative. In late, adequately treated syphilis, the serology may be fixed at a high positive titer although the patient is, in effect, cured. In late, improperly treated syphilis, the serology may be negative even though the patient is not cured and is developing central nervous system involvement.

Serological tests for syphilis are performed routinely in many situations, often because of legal requirements. For example, many states require a serological test before issuing a marriage license. Many physicians have these tests performed on all pregnant women to avoid congenital syphilis in the newborn.

Food and drink restrictions None.

Procedure for collecting specimen Collect 5 ml of *venous* blood in a collecting tube with a red stopper.

Laboratory procedure This varies with the test being performed.

Possible interfering materials and conditions In several diseases of the immune system, such as lupus erythematosus, there may be false positive serological reactions for syphilis.

There may be a false positive VDRL reaction if cetylcide, a disinfectant, comes in contact with the specimen.

Normal range Normally these tests are negative. If the reaction is faintly positive, it may denote some disorder other than syphilis.

Serum Albumin, Serum Globulin, Serum Protein *See* Albumin, Globulin, Total Protein

Serum Hepatitis Test *See* Australia Antigen Assay

Serum Transaminase

Transaminases are enzymes that catalyze the transfer of an amino grouping (NH_2) from an amino acid to an alpha keto acid. There are several different kinds of transaminases. The most commonly measured ones are the glutamic oxaloacetic transaminase (sometimes abbreviated SGOT) and the glutamic pyruvic transaminase (sometimes abbreviated SGPT). Transaminases are found normally in heart, liver, muscle, kidney, and pancreas. Elevated serum levels are seen in disease conditions in which the transaminases leak from the dead or damaged cells into the serum. Since there are several transaminases in each type of cell, there are likely to be serum elevations of more than one type of transaminase when an organ is damaged. Accordingly, there is nothing specific about elevations of serum transaminase levels. Their value in diagnosis depends on careful comparison with the results of physical examinations and other laboratory tests.

Serum Glutamic Oxaloacetic Transaminase (SGOT)

In myocardial infarction, the GOT in the heart muscle cells leaks out and increases serum levels from 4 to 10 times. The peak level is usually reached about 24 hours after infarction, and returns to normal by about the fifth day. The test is used primarily in the diagnosis of myocardial infarction.

In liver diseases, serum GOT levels may be 10 to 100 times normal and remain elevated for long periods. In the diagnosis and management of some types of liver disease, such as viral hepatitis, the level of serum GOT may provide useful information on the progress of the condition.

Food and drink restrictions   None.

Procedure for collecting specimen   Collect 5 ml of *venous* blood in a collecting tube with a red stopper. It is best to draw the blood before any drugs are given, even if at night. The enzyme in the serum is stable for about 4 days at refrigerator temperature; therefore, a specimen can be drawn at any time, allowed to clot, and then placed in the refrigerator until the laboratory can test it. The time of withdrawing the blood should be noted.

Laboratory procedure   Several methods for measuring serum GOT are available. Currently, both colorimetric and spectrophotometric measurements are in use.

Possible interfering materials and conditions   The drugs listed below can cause elevations in serum GOT levels. However, it is not yet clear whether the elevations are artifacts or whether they result from slight liver damage by the drugs that are listed here by official (generic) names only:

ampicillin	methyldopa
azaserine	morphine
carbenicillin	narcotics
chlorpromazine (information on derivatives not yet available)	oxacillin
	para-aminosalicylic acid
	pyrazinamide
codeine	pyridoxine
dicumarol	salicylates (see Table 27)
erythromycin	sulfamethoxypyridazine
ethyl biscoumacetate	vitamin B_6
iproniazid	

The ingestion of lead, even without evident poisoning, may produce elevations to 300 to 400 units.

Normal range *Adults:* Several types of unit are in use. When Karmen units are used, the normal adult range is 6 to 40 units/ml of serum. When International milliunits are used, the normal adult range is 3 to 21 milliunits/ml of serum. When International units are used, the normal adult range is 3 to 21 units/L. *Children:* In newborns, the normal level may be almost four times the normal level for adults. In other children, the normal range is similar to that for adults.

Serum Glutamic Pyruvic Transaminase (SGPT)

This enzyme, like the GOT, is found in several tissues, and its serum levels become elevated when these tissues are diseased. The serum GPT levels are used mainly in the diagnosis of liver disease. In cases of hepatitis, serum GPT rises higher than GOT levels, reaching levels of 4000 units. It falls slowly, reaching normal levels in about 2 to 3 months, unless complications occur. In cases of liver damage due to drugs and chemicals, the serum GPT levels can be even higher than in hepatitis. The major clinical value of the test appears to be in the differential diagnosis of jaundice. If the jaundice is caused by disease of the liver itself, serum GPT levels are likely to be considerably higher than 300 units. However, if the jaundice results from a condition outside the liver, the serum GPT levels are likely to be less than 300 units. In some cases comparison of serum GOT and GPT levels can give useful clues to the diagnosis, but the details of such comparisons are beyond the scope of this book.

Food and drink restrictions None.

Procedure for collecting specimen Collect 5 ml of *venous* blood in a collecting tube with a red stopper.

Laboratory procedure Several methods for determining serum GPT are available. Currently, both colorimetric and spectrophotometric measurements are in use.

Possible interfering materials and conditions Although a number of drugs and chemicals produce elevated serum GPT levels, it appears that this is not an artifact, but rather the result of toxicity affecting the liver.

The ingestion of lead, even without evident poisoning, may produce elevations to 300 to 400 units.

Normal range

Adults: 6 to 36 Karmen units/ml *or*
5 to 24 International milliunits/ml *or*
5 to 24 International units/L

Children: Similar to that for adults.

SGOT   *See* Serum Transaminase

SGPT   *See* Serum Transaminase

Sickle Cell Test

This test is performed to demonstrate an unusual type of red blood cell, which contains a different type of hemoglobin that is relatively insoluble when unoxygenated. When the available oxygen is reduced, the hemoglobin may precipitate within the cell, causing it to assume the shape of a sickle. This may interfere with the free flow of blood and cause various disorders. Most people with the sickling trait in their red cells have no demonstrable disease but may require special care and attention in surgery and obstetrics to avoid hypoxia (diminution of oxygen supply). Although the sickling trait is more often found in blacks, it may also be found in other persons.

Food and drink restrictions   None.

Procedure for collecting specimen   Collect 3 ml of *venous* blood in a collecting tube with a lavender stopper.

Laboratory procedure   A single-phase test, using a commercial kit, is commonly used.

Possible interfering materials and conditions   If the patient has received a blood transfusion within three months of the test, the results may be altered by the presence of the donor's red cells.

Normal range   Sickling is not a disease in the usual sense. There is no normal or abnormal range.

Sodium

Sodium is the main cation of the blood and extracellular fluid. Its concentration may vary within narrow limits, but if these are exceeded, serious disturbances or even death may result. Increased serum sodium levels may be found after markedly inadequate water intake and following administration of excessive amounts of sodium. Decreased sodium levels may occur in diarrhea, heat exhaustion, Addison's disease, and certain kidney disorders.

Food and drink restrictions   None.

Procedure for collecting specimen   Collect 3 ml of *venous* blood in a collecting tube with a red stopper.

Laboratory procedure   The serum concentration of sodium is measured in a flame photometer.

Possible interfering materials and conditions   None reported yet.

Normal range   *Adults:* 136 to 142 mEq/L. *Children:* Similar to that for adults.

STS   *See* Serological Tests for Syphilis

Sugar   *See* Glucose

Sulfhemoglobin

Sulfhemoglobin is not ordinarily found in the blood. It is produced when sulfides combine with the hemoglobin in the blood. It is usually associated with the intake of excessive amounts of acetanilid or phenacetin, or with hydrogen sulfide poisoning.

Food and drink restrictions   None.

Procedure for collecting specimen   Collect 5 ml of *venous* blood in a collecting tube with a green stopper.

Laboratory procedure   The blood is examined spectroscopically for the absorption bands in the transmitted light beam.

Possible interfering materials and conditions   None reported yet.

Normal range   Normally there is no sulfhemoglobin in the blood.

Sulfobromophthalein   *See* Bromsulphalein Retention

Sulfonamide Level

This test is no longer in common use in most hospital laboratories, but it may still be ordered. When treating patients with sulfonamide drugs it is often helpful to know the concentration of the drug in the blood in order to decide whether to change dosage. This test measures the concentration of sulfonamides in the blood and may be adapted to measure their concentration in any body fluid.

Food and drink restrictions   None.

Procedure for collecting specimen   Collect 5 ml of *venous* blood in a collecting tube with a green stopper.

Laboratory procedure   A colorimetric procedure is used.

Possible interfering materials and conditions   The levels of sulfonamides may be falsely elevated if the patient has been taking acetophenetidin, sometimes also called phenacetin. This drug is incorporated into many mixtures for over-the-counter and prescription sale. Most of the salicylate mixtures listed in Table 27 contain acetophenetidin.

Normal range   Normally there are no sulfonamides in the blood. The therapeutic level sought varies not only with the specific drug used but also with the invading microorganism. Some bacteria are much more sensitive to sulfonamides than others. In general, levels of between 5 and 15 mg/100 ml of serum are sought.

T3 Resin Uptake

T3 is an abbreviation for triiodothyronine, one of the two known thyroid hormones. Triiodothyronine is shorter acting but more potent than the other hormone, tetraiodothyronine (T4, thyroxine). The level of T3 in the serum is decreased in several varieties of hypothyroidism. Increased serum levels of T3 are found in hyperthyroidism.

This test is particularly useful for patients who have had iodine in medicines, diagnostic agents, food, or other substances. Such iodine can produce false and misleading results in tests based on iodine concentration. However, the T3 Resin Uptake is not affected by ordinary iodine. It can, however, be affected by radioiodine.

Food and drink restrictions   None.

Procedure for collecting specimen   Collect 5 ml of *venous* blood in a collecting tube with a red stopper.

Laboratory procedure   A sample of the patient's serum is put into a test tube containing radioactive T3 and synthetic resin particles. After an incubation period, the resin particles are washed, and the radioactivity that remains on the resin is measured.

Possible interfering materials and conditions   Previous administration of radioactive iodine to the patient may give erroneous results. If the patient has been receiving diphenylhydantoin, salicylates, oral contraceptives, or steroids, the results may be spuriously low. If the patient has been on heparin or oral anticoagulants, the results may be spuriously high.

Normal range   *Adults:* This depends on the type of resin used. If the common one, Triosorb, is used, the normal range is 25 to 35%. *Children:* The normal range has not been established.

T4   *See* Thyroxine

TG   *See* Triglycerides

Thymol Turbidity

This liver function test is gradually being replaced by more specific tests. Normally, when serum is mixed with a saturated solution of thymol, turbidity is seen. The turbidity is usually increased in liver conditions, such as hepatitis, in which the liver cells are damaged. In biliary obstruction without damage to the liver cells, the turbidity is usually normal.

Food and drink restrictions   The patient must avoid foods and beverages containing fat (including milk) for at least 12 hours before the blood sample is drawn. Water may be taken freely.

Procedure for collecting specimen   Collect 5 ml of *venous* blood in a collecting tube with a red stopper.

Laboratory procedure   A sample of serum is added to a saturated solution of thymol. The degree of turbidity produced is measured colorimetrically or by comparison with a set of standards.

Possible interfering materials and conditions   The thymol turbidity reading may be increased by lipemia. Therefore, the patient should avoid fatty foods for at least 12 hours before blood is drawn for the test. Unfortunately, the usual hospital diet is high in fats, so that fasting may be necessary.

Normal range *Adults:* Fewer than 5 units. *Children:* This test is not commonly performed on children.

Thyroid Antibodies

In certain diseases, known as autoimmune diseases, the causative organism produces antibodies that attack normal tissues. One example is Hashimoto's thyroiditis, in which antibodies to the thyroid gland are produced. The antibodies attack the normal cells and also combine with the thyroglobulin produced by the thyroid. A measurement of the titer of these antibodies is helpful in the diagnosis of Hashimoto's disease, although such antibodies are sometimes found in other conditions and in a few healthy persons.

Food and drink restrictions None.

Procedure for collecting specimen Collect 5 ml of *venous* blood in a collecting tube with a red stopper.

Laboratory procedure Usually, the ability of the patient's serum to agglutinate latex particles coated with thyroglobulin is measured.

Possible interfering materials and conditions Other types of thyroid disease may also result in production of thyroid antibodies.

Normal range *Adults:* About 6 to 10% of normal adults may have some detectable thyroid antibodies. *Children:* This test is not usually performed on children and normal standards have not been established.

Thyroid-Stimulating Hormone (TSH)

The thyroid-stimulating hormone, which is produced by the pituitary gland, stimulates the thyroid to produce thyroxine. When there is a deficiency in thyroid function (hypothyroidism), it is important to know whether the deficiency exists because the thyroid is not responding to the pituitary stimulation or because the pituitary stimulation is defective.

The levels of thyroid-stimulating hormone and of thyroxine can usually point to the basis of the problem. In hypothyroidism, decreased thyroxine levels with normal or elevated levels of thyroid-stimulating hormone suggest that the primary disorder is in the thyroid. On the other hand, decreased thyroxine levels with decreased levels of thyroid-stimulating hormone suggest a primary lesion in the pituitary.

In cases of hyperthyroidism, measurement of thyroid-stimulating hormone levels is not as yet particularly useful.

Food and drink restrictions None.

Procedure for collecting specimen Collect 5 ml of *venous* blood in a collecting tube with a red stopper.

Laboratory procedure A radioimmunoassay procedure is often used.

Possible interfering materials and conditions None reported yet.

Normal range *Adults:* This depends on the laboratory. A representative level is up to 0.2 mμ/ml of serum. *Children:* This test has not been done long enough for normal levels to be established.

Thyrotropin *See* Thyroid-Stimulating Hormone

Thyroxine (T4)

This test for the serum level of the main thyroid hormone is a more specific test of thyroid function than the older protein-bound iodine test, and less subject to interference. However, it appears to be a more complex test, and there is still wide discrepancy between the normal ranges used by various hospital laboratories. Elevation of thyroxine levels is found in hyperthyroidism, and depression of thyroxine levels is found in hypothyroidism.

Food and drink restrictions None.

Procedure for collecting specimen Collect 5 ml of *venous* blood in a collecting tube with a red stopper.

Laboratory procedure Several procedures are available.

Possible interfering materials and conditions Patients who are seriously ill with diseases not directly involving the thyroid often have high thyroxine levels.

Diphenylhydantoin (Dilantin) and related drugs may interfere with the test results, giving spuriously low values, depending on the laboratory procedures used. Oral contraceptives may give high values, but these may be true values caused by the pharmacologic action of the drug.

Normal range   The normal range varies considerably depending on the procedure used and on the particular techniques in each laboratory. Accordingly, a generally accepted normal range cannot as yet be given.

Total Cholesterol   *See* Cholesterol

Total Protein   *See* Albumin, Globulin, Total Protein

TPI   *See* Treponemal Immobilization Test

Transaminase   *See* Serum Transaminase, Serum Glutamic Oxaloacetic Transaminase (SGOT), and Glutamic Pyruvic Transaminase (SGPT)

Triglycerides (TG)

Triglycerides are fats. Their level in the blood varies considerably depending on the time that has elapsed since the last meal. If the patient has been fasting for at least 12 hours before the blood sample is drawn, the triglyceride level should normally be quite low. If it is elevated, however, one of several disorders of fat metabolism may be present. These disorders are usually referred to collectively as hyperlipoproteinemias. In the past, many terms were used for these disorders. More recently, the World Health Organization has classified hyperlipoproteinemias by Roman numerals I through V. In types I, III, IV, and V, the fasting triglyceride level is usually elevated. In type II, it may be normal or elevated. Many disorders of metabolism are associated with hyperlipoproteinemias. It is not always clear which came first. Examples of other disorders associated with hyperlipoproteinemias include alcoholism, diabetes, dysglobulinemias, autoimmune disorders, glycogen storage disease, hypothyroidism, nephrosis, and pancreatitis.

By itself, an elevated fasting triglyceride level indicates merely that something is wrong. Other tests are needed to determine exactly which disorder is present. The triglyceride level is commonly measured together with cholesterol levels. The relationship between the two often gives a clue to the diagnosis.

Food and drink restrictions   For two weeks before the test, the patient should adhere to a diet that would be considered usual for people living in the United States. On the day before the test, the last meal should be no later than 6:00 p.m. and should not include excessive fat. Water may be taken freely.

Procedure for collecting specimen   Collect 5 ml of *venous* blood in a collecting tube with a red stopper.

Laboratory procedure   Several procedures are available.

Possible interfering materials and conditions   It appears probable that several drugs can affect the serum triglyceride levels, but which drugs have this effect is not yet definitely known. Accordingly, it is advisable to discontinue almost all drugs, including nonprescription items, for at least 24 hours before the serum sample is drawn. This may not always be possible as, for example, in cases of severe diabetes.

Normal range   *Adults:* 10 to 190 mg/100 ml. Some hospitals have a maximum limit of normality as low as 135 mg/100 ml, depending on the procedure used. *Children:* This test is not commonly done on children and normal values have not been definitely established.

Triiodothyronine Resin Uptake   *See* T3 Resin Uptake

TSH   *See* Thyroid-Stimulating Hormone

Unsaturated Iron-Binding Capacity   *See* Iron-Binding Capacity

Urea Clearance   *See* Urea Clearance, Chapter 5

Urea Nitrogen—Blood Urea Nitrogen (BUN)

This is a test of kidney function. Ordinarily the kidney readily excretes urea, the end product of protein metabolism, so that the blood urea concentration is fairly low. However, in certain kidney disorders the ability to excrete urea may be impaired, so that the concentration of urea nitrogen in the blood increases. This test gives essentially the same information as the nonprotein nitrogen (NPN) test and is somewhat more accurate. There is no reason to do both tests, and therefore, in most laboratories one or the other is performed. A rising blood urea nitrogen level may portend mental clouding, confusion, and disorientation, and the patient may eventually go into coma. Therefore, when the laboratory report indicates a rising blood urea nitrogen content, the nurse should be prepared to deal with a patient who might become difficult to handle.

Food and drink restrictions   None.

Procedure for collecting specimen   Collect 5 ml of *venous* blood in a collecting tube with a red stopper.

Laboratory procedure   The urea is converted to ammonia by the enzyme urease. The amount of ammonia is then measured photometrically.

Possible interfering materials and conditions   Many substances may cause elevations in the blood urea nitrogen concentrations. In most cases the elevation is real, caused by a drug effect on the kidney, but this is a transient effect, and the level returns to normal soon after the drug is discontinued. Therefore, an elevation in blood urea nitrogen in patients receiving such drugs may not indicate preexisting kidney disease. The drugs, listed mainly by official (generic) name, include:

acetohexamide	gentamycin
amphotericin B	guanethidine
antimony compounds	Guanochlor
arsenicals	indomethacin
bacitracin	kanamycin
blood, whole	Lipomul
capreomycin	methicillin
cephaloridine (high doses)	methyldopa
chloral hydrate (see	methysergide
Table 19)	nalidixic acid
chlorthalidone	neomycin
colistimethate	pargyline
doxapram	polymyxin B
ethacrynic acid	radiopaque contrast media
furosemide	(see Table 22 B)

salicylates (see Table 27)   thiazides
streptokinase-   triamterene
  streptodornase   vancomycin

Normal range   *Adults:* 9 to 20 mg of urea *nitrogen*/100 ml of blood. The amount of actual urea, as distinct from urea nitrogen, ranges from 19 to 40 mg/100 ml of blood, but this value is seldom mentioned clinically. *Children:* Similar to or slightly lower than the range for adults.

Uric Acid

This test is usually performed to diagnose gout, but it may also give significant results in other conditions. Uric acid is the end product of purine metabolism, and purines come mainly from cell nuclei. The blood uric acid concentration in gout is high. The reason for this is unknown. The uric acid concentration may also be elevated in conditions involving marked cellular destruction, such as leukemia, pneumonia, and toxemias of pregnancy. When kidney damage is severe, there may be an elevated uric acid level because of decreased excretion. However, such an elevation does not afford an accurate index of kidney function.

Food and drink restrictions   None.

Procedure for collecting specimen   Collect 5 ml of *venous* blood in a collecting tube with a red stopper.

Laboratory procedure   A colorimetric method is commonly used.

Possible interfering materials and conditions   The uric acid levels may be elevated by several drugs and treatments. Listed by official (generic) name these include:

ascorbic acid   pyrazinamide
blood transfusions   salicylates (see Table 27)
chlorothiazide   theophylline
nitrogen mustards   thiazides

The levels may be lowered by coumarin anticoagulants and piperazine.

Normal range

Adults: Male: 2 to 7.8 mg / 100 ml
             Female: 2 to 6.5 mg / 100 ml

Children: Newborn to 15 years: 2.2 to 5.3 mg/100 ml
              After 15 years: adult range applies

Van den Bergh Test   *See* Bilirubin, Partition

VDRL   *See* Serological Tests for Syphilis

Wassermann   *See* Serological Tests for Syphilis

White Cell Count   *See* Blood Counts, White Cell Count

White Cell Differential Count   *See* Blood Counts, White Cell
    Differential Count

Zinc Sulfate Turbidity

This test of liver function has been replaced by more specific tests
including those for determining immunoglobulin levels.

4

Tests Performed
on Cerebrospinal Fluid (CSF)

Cerebrospinal fluid, often called spinal fluid, fills the ventricles of the brain and the central canal of the spinal cord. It acts as a fluid buffer that can enlarge or diminish in volume, when necessary, to protect the brain and spinal cord from compression injury when slight changes occur in the volume of the space enclosed by the cranium and spinal column. It may also help prevent traumatic jarring of the brain. The cerebrospinal fluid may also play a role in supplying oxygen and nutrients to the brain and cord and in removing waste.

Cerebrospinal fluid is produced from blood by the choroid plexus, a highly vascular structure in the brain ventricles. CSF differs from filtrate of blood in several respects, and the exact mechanism by which it is formed is not known. It is, however, in osmotic equilibrium with the blood.

From the brain ventricles where it is produced, the cerebrospinal fluid passes slowly down the spinal canal and is slowly reabsorbed into the blood. Approximately 100 ml of cerebrospinal fluid is normally present and usually that amount is produced and reabsorbed daily.

Because of its intimate association with the brain and spinal cord, cerebrospinal fluid is a useful indicator of disease in those organs.

Usually, cerebrospinal fluid is obtained by lumbar puncture. In this procedure the physician withdraws fluid after passing a needle between two lumbar vertebrae into the spinal canal. Lumbar puncture is to be viewed as the equivalent of a surgical operation. The same sterile precautions are essential. In some institutions the patient must sign a permission form before lumbar puncture can be performed.

Occasionally, the cerebrospinal fluid is obtained by puncture of the cisterna magna. This requires insertion of a needle between the base of the skull and the first cervical vertebra. It can be done safely by physicians specially trained in this technique.

After the needle has entered the spinal canal, the physician usually performs several tests of the cerebrospinal fluid pressure. Only after these have been done are fluid samples withdrawn for laboratory examination. The fluid samples are not placed in a single container, but into a series of small test tubes, usually 3 or 4, depending on the tests ordered. The test tubes must be kept in the correct order, since the first tubes are more likely to contain minute amounts of blood from the puncture. Tests that would be affected by small amounts of blood are therefore performed on fluid contained in the last tubes.

Cell Count (Leukocyte)

This test often indicates the presence of infection, such as meningitis. It is usually performed immediately following lumbar puncture and requires only about 15 minutes. The cell count is moderately increased (10 to 200 per cu mm) in such conditions as poliomyelitis, encephalitis, and neurosyphilis. Cell counts of several thousand per cu mm are found in most cases of meningitis.

Food and drink restrictions None.

Procedure for collecting specimen The physician places 1 to 2 ml of cerebrospinal fluid in a special small test tube. Usually the third tube in the series is used, since it is less likely to contain minute amounts of blood.

Laboratory procedure A hemocytometer counting chamber, which is placed under the microscope, is used for making the count.

Possible interfering materials and conditions None reported yet.

Normal range 0 to 8 cells/cu mm.

Chlorides

The cerebrospinal fluid chlorides are reduced in some types of meningitis, particularly tuberculous meningitis. Measurement of the chloride level may aid in differential diagnosis.

Food and drink restrictions None.

Procedure for collecting specimen   The physician places 2 ml of cerebrospinal fluid in a special small test tube.

Laboratory procedure   The same as for blood chlorides.

Possible interfering materials and conditions   None reported yet.

Normal range   *Adults:* 118 to 133 mEq/L. *Children:* 120-128 mEq/L.

Colloidal Gold

This test is no longer in common use, since better methods of diagnosis are now available.

Culture   *See* Spinal Fluid Culture, Chapter 2

Protein

The spinal fluid protein is increased in several diseases of the central nervous system, especially meningitis and subarachnoid hemorrhage. Qualitative tests are now being replaced with simple quantitative tests of greater accuracy.

Food and drink restrictions   None.

Procedure for collecting specimen   The physician places 2 ml of cerebrospinal fluid in a special small test tube. The last test tube of cerebrospinal fluid collected should be used for protein determination.

Laboratory procedure   Several different procedures are available.

Possible interfering materials and conditions   The spinal fluid protein level can appear falsely elevated by several drugs, if the measurement involves the use of the phosphomolybdic-phosphotungstic acid reagent (Folin-Ciocalteau reagent). Drugs that may have this effect are listed below by their official or their common name:

acetophenetidin   chlorpromazine
aspirin   (Thorazine)

many drugs for mild pain relief	salicylates (see Table 27)
many headache remedies	streptomycin
phenacetin	sulfonamides

If any local anesthetic gets into the spinal canal, this too will produce a spurious elevation of the cerebrospinal fluid protein when the Folin-Ciocalteau reagent is used.

Normal range   *Adults:* 15 to 45 mg/100 ml. *Children:* Same as the range for adults.

Serological Tests

These tests are performed to discover the presence of neurosyphilis. A positive serological reaction of the spinal fluid almost always indicates neurosyphilis.

Food and drink restrictions   None.

Procedure for collecting specimen   The physician places 7 ml of spinal fluid in a small test tube.

Laboratory procedure   A serologic test is performed, similar to that done on blood.

Possible interfering materials and conditions   None reported yet.

Normal range   Normally the serological reaction is negative.

Sugar

Spinal fluid sugar is decreased in meningitis. This test is often useful in the differential diagnosis of central nervous system conditions.

Food and drink restrictions   None.

Procedure for collecting specimen   The physician places 2 ml of cerebrospinal fluid in a special small test tube. If the test cannot be performed at once, breakdown of sugar must be prevented by preservation with a thymol crystal.

Laboratory procedure   A colorimetric method is used.

Possible interfering materials and conditions   None reported yet.

Normal range   *Adults:* 45 to 75 mg/100 ml. *Children:* 35 to 75 mg/100 ml.

5

Tests Performed on Urine

Urine is formed by the kidneys. The glomeruli of the kidneys allow a filtrate of the blood plasma to pass into the tubules. The tubule cells may also excrete certain substances into the urine being formed. During a 24-hour period, a total of about 200 liters of fluid is filtered through the glomeruli and about 199 liters are reabsorbed by the tubules. The difference represents the urine excreted.

Although it is believed that the primary function of the kidneys is the excretion of wastes, other functions are as important if not more so. They include regulation of ionic balance, acid-base balance, and water balance of the body. Urine will vary widely in composition from time to time. Such variations are not abnormal, but are indicative of good function.

Some authorities divide tests of kidney function into three groups: those that test glomerular filtration (e.g., urea clearance), those that test tubular reabsorption (e.g., concentration and dilution tests), and those that test the excretion by the tubules (e.g., phenolsulfonphthalein excretion tests). Many kidney disorders, however, may involve both glomeruli and tubules, so that interpretation of the results of these tests requires considerable skill and experience. There are also many tests of urine that are done to evaluate the condition of organs other than the kidney.

Urine preservatives Urine specimens that cannot be sent directly to the laboratory should be protected against bacterial decomposition, which can invalidate or confuse test results. This includes all 24-hour urine specimens. In general, refrigeration is an important method of preserving urine for short periods. In collecting 24-hour specimens, one should *not* leave the large urine bottle at the patient's bedside. Instead, the large container should be kept in the refrigerator, and each voiding of urine during the 24-hour interval should be collected in fresh, clean, smaller containers that are then emptied promptly into the large refrigerated bottle.

For some tests, it is also appropriate to use a chemical in order to reduce bacterial proliferation. In general, 10 ml of toluene or 1 ml of *glacial* acetic acid will preserve a liter of urine. However, for some tests, special preservatives are needed, since toluene or acetic acid would invalidate the results.

Aceto-Acetic Acid   *See* Ketone Bodies, Urine

Acetone   *See* Ketone Bodies, Urine

Albumin, Qualitative

Ordinarily the albumin in the blood does not pass through the glomerular wall into the urine. However, in such conditions as kidney disease, hypertension, severe heart failure, or drug toxicity, albumin appears in the urine. It may also be seen in orthostatic albuminuria, which is not a disease. Therefore, the test is not specific, but a positive reaction indicates that more precise tests are needed.

Food and drink restrictions   None.

Procedure for collecting specimen   A urine specimen is placed in a bottle and sent to the laboratory.

Laboratory procedure   There are several procedures in use. A popular test uses a plastic strip.

Possible interfering materials and conditions   Many drugs are capable of producing a positive test for urine albumin. Some of these test results may be spurious; others may represent a small transient amount of kidney dysfunction. Because the number of drugs having this effect is so large, it is impractical to try to include the brand names; therefore, only the official (generic) or the common names are listed here:

aminophylline	capreomycin
aminosalicylic acid	carbarsone
amphotericin B	carbutamide
antimony compounds	carinamide
arsenicals	chlorpropamide
bacitracin	colistimethate
bismuth triglycollamate	diatrizoate (may produce

4+ levels)
dihydrotachysterol
dithiazanine
doxapram
edathamil
ethosuximide
gentamycin
gold salts
griseofulvin
iodoalphionic acid
iodopanoic acid
isoniazid
kanamycin
mefenamic acid
metahexamide
metaxalone
methenamine (large doses)
methicillin
methsuximide
neomycin
paraldehyde

paramethadione
para-aminosalicylic acid
penicillamine
penicillin (large doses)
phenacemide
phenindione
polymyxin B
pyrazolone derivatives
radiographic contrast
    media (may produce
    4+ levels)
salicylates (see Table 27)
sulfisoxazole
sulfones
suramin
thiosemicarbazones
tolbutamide
trimethadione
viomycin
vitamin D

Normal range   In 5 to 15% of normal individuals small amounts of albumin are sometimes found in the urine when no disease is present. This has been termed orthostatic or postural albuminuria.

Albumin, Quantitative

This test is performed to discover the amount of albumin lost daily in the urine. This information may be helpful in attempting to restore protein balance.

Food and drink restrictions   None.

Procedure for collecting specimen   The urine excreted during a 24-hour period is collected in a clean bottle, which is kept in a refrigerator during the collection period.

Laboratory procedure   Several methods may be used, all of which involve the addition of reagents that precipitate the albumin. The amount of precipitate or degree of turbidity is then compared to standards.

Possible interfering materials and conditions   Many drugs are capable of producing a positive test for urine albumin. Some of these test results may be spurious; others may represent a small transient amount of kidney dysfunction. Because the number of drugs having this effect is so large, it is impractical to try to include the brand names, and therefore only the official or the common names are listed here:

aminophylline
aminosalicylic acid
amphotericin B
antimony compounds
arsenicals
bacitracin
bismuth triglycollamate
capreomycin
carbarsone
carbutamide
carinamide
chlorpropamide
colistimethate
diatrizoate (may produce
   4+ levels)
dihydrotachysterol
dithiazanine
doxapram
edathamil
ethosuximide
gentamycin
gold salts
griseofulvin
iodoalphionic acid
iodopanoic acid
isoniazid
kanamycin
mefenamic acid

metahexamide
metaxalone
methenamine (large doses)
methicillin
methsuximide
neomycin
paraldehyde
paramethadione
para-aminosalicylic acid
penicillamine
penicillin (large doses)
phenacemide
phenindione
polymyxin B
pyrazolone derivatives
radiographic contrast
   media (may produce
   4+ levels)
salicylates (see Table 27)
sulfisoxazole
sulfones
suramin
thiosemicarbazones
tolbutamide
trimethadione
viomycin
vitamin D

Normal range   In 5 to 15% of normal individuals small amounts of albumin are sometimes found in the urine when no disease is present. This has been termed orthostatic or postural albuminuria.

Amino Acids

This series of tests for excess of particular amino acids in the urine is used to determine whether one or another type of condition, often congenital in nature, may be present. Two main types of conditions lead to excess amino acids in the urine. The so-called renal type results from a defect in the renal tubules. In some defects—for example, the Fanconi syndrome—all amino acids are excreted in the urine in increased amounts. In other renal tubular defects, there may be an increased excretion of all or some amino acids, but a much greater excretion of one or more particular amino acids. When the aminoaciduria is caused by a defect in the renal tubule, the plasma levels of the amino acids are generally normal.

The second type of aminoaciduria is called the "overflow" type. In this condition, abnormal metabolism of one or more amino acids leads to an extremely high level in the plasma, so that normal tubular reabsorption cannot handle the load, and some spills over into the urine. Many of these overflow aminoacidurias are caused by congenital metabolic defects. Phenylketonuria is perhaps the best-known example.

Chromatography and electrophoresis are employed whenever aminoaciduria is suspected, and the results of the test generally indicate the kinds of amino acids being excreted in excess. They do not, however, distinguish between renal and overflow types. To make that distinction, studies of the plasma are also needed.

In some cases, additional tests are applicable to specific types of aminoaciduria.

Many diverse conditions can cause aminoaciduria, including congenital disorders, heavy metal and other types of poisoning, severe burns, and liver and kidney diseases. The major causes of aminoaciduria are summarized in the table on pp. 132–133.

Food and drink restrictions   None reported.

Procedure for collecting specimen   Usually a fresh urine specimen is needed, although in some hospitals a 24-hour specimen may be required. This test is frequently performed on infants, and particular care must be exercised to prevent any contamination of the urine by feces.

Laboratory procedure   The amino acids are identified in the urine by high-voltage paper electrophoresis and paper chromatography.

MAIN TYPES OF AMINOACIDURIA

Disease	Type of Disease	Mechanism of Aminoaciduria	Amino Acids in Excess in Urine
alkaptonuria	congenital	overflow	homogentisic acid
aminoaciduria of liver disease	acquired	overflow	all
argininosuccinic aciduria	congenital	overflow	argininosuccinic acid, citrulline
burns, severe	acquired	renal	several
citrullinemia	congenital	overflow	citrulline
cystathioninuria	congenital	overflow	cystathionine
cystinuria	congenital	renal	cystine, lysine, arginine, ornithine
Fanconi syndrome	acquired	renal	several
fructose intolerance	congenital	renal	several
galactosemia	congenital	renal	all
glycinuria	congenital	renal	glycine
Hartnup disease	congenital	renal	most
heavy metal poisoning	acquired	renal	several
histidinemia	congenital	overflow	histidine
hemocystinuria	congenital	overflow	methionine, hemocystine
hydroxyprolinemia	congenital	overflow	hydroxyproline
hyperglycinemia	congenital	overflow	glycine, and sometimes leucine
hyperlysinemia	congenital	overflow	lysine
hyperprolinemia	congenital	overflow	proline
hypervalinemia	congenital	overflow	valine
hypophosphatasia	congenital	overflow	phosphoethanolamine
maleic acid poisoning	acquired	renal	several
maple-syrup urine disease	congenital	overflow	valine, leucine and isoleucine
Oasthouse urine disease	congenital	overflow	phenylalanine, methionine, valine, leucine, isoleucine, and tyrosine
oxalic acid poisoning	acquired	renal	several
phenol poisoning	acquired	renal	several
phenylketonuria	congenital	overflow	phenylalanine
rickets	acquired	renal	several
scurvy	acquired	renal	several

Disease	Type of Disease	Mechanism of Aminoaciduria	Amino Acids in Excess in Urine
starvation	acquired	overflow	beta-amino-isobutyric acid
tyrosinosis	congenital	overflow	tyrosine
von Gierke's disease	congenital	renal	several
Wilson's disease	congenital	renal	all

Possible interfering materials and conditions   The screening test for homogentisic acid (p. 148) may produce a false positive result if the patient has received salicylates (Table 27) in the preceding 3 days. However, the chromatographic test should give accurate results.

The screening test for phenylketonuria (p. 162) may be interfered with if the patient has received phenothiazines (Table 25), or salicylates (Table 27). However, the chromatographic test should give accurate results.

If protein hydrolysate is given intravenously, there will be a generalized aminoaciduria.

Normal range   *Adults:* A normal adult excretes from 300 to 650 mg of amino acids in the urine every 24 hours. This contains from 50 to 200 mg of amino acid nitrogen. The relative concentrations of the different amino acids vary somewhat, and are seldom measured directly. Abnormalities are detected by comparing the test chromatogram with a normal pattern. *Children:* This depends to some extent on the type and frequency of feeding. Normally, large amounts of taurine are present at birth but reach adult levels at 6 months.

Aminolevulinic Acid (ALA)

This is a sensitive test for diagnosing clinically significant overexposure to lead. It often becomes positive before any symptoms are observable.

Food and drink restrictions   None.

Procedure for collecting specimen   A urine specimen is collected and sent to the laboratory immediately. If the test is not done at once, the specimen must be protected from light, acidified with glacial acetic acid or hydrochloric acid, and refrigerated. Sometimes a 24-hour specimen is needed.

Laboratory procedure   Procedures are in the process of refinement.

Possible interfering materials and methods   None reported yet.

Normal range   *Adults:* This is not yet agreed upon. Some authorities consider normal to be any level below 5 mg in 24 hours, other consider 7.5 mg in 24 hours to be the upper limit of normal. For a random urine specimen, the upper limit of normal is about 0.6 mg/100 ml. *Children:* At 1 year of age and over, the normal range is probably similar to that for adults. The normal range for infants under 1 year is not yet established.

Amylase   *See* Amylase, Chapter 3

This is a test for pancreatic diseases in which the digestive enzymes of the pancreas may escape into the surrounding tissue, producing necrosis with severe pain and inflammation. These enzymes, including amylase, are found in the serum, where they can be measured (see p. 28), and are excreted in the urine. The serum amylase levels tend to remain high for a short time, sometimes only a few hours, while the urine levels remain high for about a week. Therefore, when the physician suspects that the time for finding the elevated serum amylase level might have passed, he may order a urinary amylase determination.

Food and drink restrictions   None.

Procedure for collecting specimen   A timed collection is required. Institutions vary as to the time intervals used. Some use a 2-hour specimen, others a 12- or 24-hour specimen. It is essential that the exact times of the beginning and the end of the collection period be recorded and sent to the laboratory with the specimen. The *beginning* of a collection period is the time when a patient empties his bladder, with that specimen being discarded. All subsequent urine specimens are saved, including the one at the end of the collection period.

It is not clear which, if any, preservatives are suitable for these urine specimens and which might interfere with the test. Unless the laboratory specifies that a preservative may be used, it would be best to avoid the preservative and keep the urine sample refrigerated until it is sent to the laboratory.

Laboratory procedure   Starch in solution is hydrolysed by the urinary amylase. At intervals, aliquots are tested with iodine solution and the times at which color changes occur are compared to standards.

Possible interfering materials and conditions   The data on possible interfering materials and conditions for urinary amylase measurements and interpretations is incomplete and unclear. It seems prudent to assume that materials and conditions that interfere with *serum* amylase level interpretations may likewise interfere with urinary level interpretations.

The following drugs, therefore, might produce elevations of urinary amylase levels:

bethanechol (Urecholine, Myocholine)
codeine
ethyl alcohol (large amounts)

meperidine (Demerol)
methyl alcohol (large amounts)
morphine
narcotic drugs

There may be a spurious decrease in apparent urinary amylase levels if the urine specimens become contaminated with fluorides.

The following conditions may produce elevated urinary amylase levels:

mumps
diseases of salivary glands and ducts
some intestinal obstructions

Any contamination of the urinary specimen by saliva may result in a spuriously high urinary amylase level. Such contamination might come from improper pipetting, or from spitting, coughing, sneezing, or even talking near the uncovered specimen.

Normal range   *Adults:* The normal range is under 270 units *per hour. Children:* This test is not commonly performed on children and the normal range is not definitely established. It is probably similar to the adult range if corrected for the relative size of the child.

Aschheim-Zondek Test

This test for pregnancy was once widely used but has now been largely replaced by simpler, less time-consuming tests.

Ascorbic Acid (Vitamin C) Tolerance (Urine)   *See also* Ascorbic Acid Tolerance (Blood)

This test measures the degree of ascorbic acid deficiency. Although not as widely performed as it once was, it can provide important clinical information. We recognize now that some persons who are on seemingly adequate diets, and even some who are receiving supplemental vitamins, may have a partial deficiency in ascorbic acid. This may occur in patients with severe burns, infection, or malignancy. A partial deficiency of ascorbic acid can interfere with wound healing, body defenses, and recovery.

When a large dose of ascorbic acid is given intravenously to normal persons, about 30% or more will be excreted in the urine. In cases of relative ascorbic acid deficiency, much less will be excreted.

Food and drink restrictions   For 24 hours before the test, the patient must avoid foods high in ascorbic acid. Water may be taken as desired.

Procedure for collecting specimen   In recent years, the procedure has been simplified so that a 5- or 6-hour urine specimen is now used instead of a 24-hour specimen. The patient empties his bladder, and this specimen is discarded. All subsequent specimens are collected in a bottle containing glacial acetic acid.

The patient receives the ascorbic acid orally or intravenously. In the oral method, 11 mg/kg of body weight is dissolved in a glass of water and swallowed. All urine voided during the next 6 hours (5 in some situations) is collected in the bottle with acetic acid and sent immediately to the laboratory at the end of the period.

In the intravenous method, the physician injects the test dose, which varies from 500 mg to 1 gm, mixed in an appropriate solution. All urine specimens during the next 5 hours are collected and sent immediately to the laboratory at the end of the period.

This test may be done in conjunction with the blood test (p. 32).

Laboratory procedure   The amount of ascorbic acid in the urine is measured photometrically after chemical modification.

Possible interfering materials and conditions   None reported yet.

Normal range   *Adults:* For the oral test—excretion of 10% of the administered amount. For the intravenous test—excretion of 30 to 40% of the administered amount. *Children:* This test is not usually performed on children.

Bacterial Count

The primary use of bacterial count of the urine is to distinguish between true infection of the urinary tract and contamination of specimens by bacteria residing near the urethral opening. In the past, catheterization was used to get urine specimens that were supposedly free of contamination. However, the disclosure that catheterization has a substantial risk (around 5%) of producing a urinary tract infection where none existed before has made it prudent to avoid catheterization. The techniques used to obtain urine specimens for culture may permit skin bacteria to contaminate the culture, but a count of the bacteria can usually reveal whether they came from an infection or from the skin. Urine bacteria counts of over 100,000/ml of urine generally mean that there is a significant urinary tract infection. Counts of less than 10,000 bacteria generally signify contamination of the sample, without true infection of the urinary tract. Counts between 10,000 and 100,000/ml of urine are inconclusive and should be repeated.

In some circumstances, bacterial counts might be used to follow the course of a patient being treated for a known urinary tract infection.

Food and drink restrictions None.

Procedure for collecting specimen One of the crucial aspects of this test is the need to minimize any delay between the collection of the specimen and the delivery to the laboratory.

To collect a specimen from a male patient, the patient starts to urinate, and then a mid-stream sample of urine is caught in a sterile container.

To collect a specimen from a female patient, the entire vulvar area is first cleaned carefully, using a dilute solution of benzalkonium (Zephiran) or hexachlorophene. Both should not be used on the same patient, however. Then, the cleaned area is rinsed with sterile water, being careful not to allow the water to flow from uncleaned to cleaned areas. Drying should be done by gentle patting with a sterile towel. Next, the labia are held apart, and after some urine has been passed, a sterile bottle is placed in the stream to catch a specimen. Specimens must then be taken to the laboratory at once.

Laboratory procedure A measured sample of the urine is plated out on culture media, and the number of bacterial colonies growing on a predetermined area of the media is counted. Since each colony arises from a single bacterium, it is possible to calculate the number of bacteria in a ml of urine.

Possible interfering materials and conditions   Any antibiotic or chemotherapeutic agents taken by the patient may interfere with the count. If the benzalkonium or hexachlorophene is not rinsed off thoroughly, and contaminates the urine sample, spuriously low readings may be obtained.

Normal range   *Adults:* Any counts under 10,000/ml of urine may be considered normal, and as resulting from external contamination. *Children:* Same as the range for adults.

Bence Jones Protein

This is a test for certain tumors. Bence Jones protein is an unusual type of protein molecule with a molecular weight of about 35,000 as compared to 70,000 for albumin. It coagulates on heating at about 45° C and redissolves at about 100° C. It is excreted in large amounts in the urine in most cases of multiple myeloma. It may also be found in other types of bone tumors.

Food and drink restrictions   None.

Procedure for collecting specimen   A urine sample is placed in a bottle and sent to the laboratory.

Laboratory procedure   The urine sample is acidified to pH 5 and heated to 45° to 70° C. If coagulation of protein is seen, the urine is heated to 100° C. If the coagulum is due to Bence Jones protein, it redissolves at 100° C and recoagulates at 70° C or less.

Possible interfering materials and conditions   Bence Jones protein may appear in the urine of patients who have taken out-dated tetracycline. It may also appear in the urine of patients with Waldenströms macroglobulinemia.

Normal range   Normally, small amounts of Bence Jones protein may be found in the urine when highly sensitive techniques are used, but the amount is too small to be observed with usual techniques in the absence of disease.

Bile and Bilirubin

This liver function test is now performed less frequently than in the past. Bile pigments and acids are found in the urine when there is obstruction of the biliary tract. Bilirubin (the main pigment) is found alone when there is excessive hemolysis of the red blood cells.

Food and drink restrictions   None.

Procedure for collecting specimen   A urine specimen is placed in a bottle and sent to the laboratory. The test for bile acids cannot be performed if the urine specimen has been preserved with thymol.

Laboratory procedure   Several tests are available. One of the most widely used employs prepackaged test tablets.

Possible interfering materials and conditions   There may be a false positive reaction for bile if the patient has taken chlorzoxazone (Paraflex).

There may be an elevation of urine bilirubin if the patient has received certain drugs. The elevation may be due to transient interference with liver function, and does not indicate permanent liver disease. These drugs, listed by official (generic) names, include:

> acetophenazine
> chlorprothixene
> ethoxazene
> phenazopyridine
> phenothiazines, some

Normal range   Bile acids and bilirubin are not normally found in the urine.

Blood

Blood in the urine may appear as intact red blood cells (hematuria) or dissolved hemoglobin derived from destroyed red blood cells (hemoglobinuria). Hematuria comes from bleeding somewhere along the urinary tract from glomerulus to urethra. The site of bleeding and its cause are determined by more precise testing methods. Hemoglobinuria usually arises from conditions outside the urinary tract. The red cells are hemolyzed and the dissolved hemoglobin in the plasma is excreted by the kidney. It is seen in severe burns, transfusion reactions, severe malaria (blackwater fever), poisoning, and paroxysmal hemoglobinuria.

Food and drink restrictions None.

Procedure for collecting specimen A urine specimen is placed in a bottle and sent to the laboratory.

Laboratory procedure Intact red blood cells are identified by centrifuging the urine and examining the sediment microscopically.

Hemoglobin is now identified by special paper strips impregnated with orthotolidine (Hemostix).

Possible interfering materials and conditions A positive test may result from myoglobin in the urine, or from large amounts of bacteria or of pus in the urine.

A false negative reaction can result when a patient receives large amounts of ascorbic acid, either as therapeutic vitamin supplements or as parenteral tetracyclines in which ascorbic acid is used as a preservative.

A large number of drugs may cause enough urinary bleeding to produce a positive reaction for blood in the urine. Although this is a true result, it can be misleading if the causative role of the drug is not understood. This bleeding does not indicate any basic urinary tract disease, and does not warrant extensive diagnostic studies. When the drug is withdrawn, the bleeding soon stops. Drugs that may cause such bleeding, listed by official (generic) name, include:

aminosalicylic acid	oxyphenbutazone
amphotericin B	methicillin
bacitracin	para-aminosalicylic acid
chloroguanide	phenindione derivatives
colchicine	phenylbutazone
corticosteroids	phytonadione
coumarin anticoagulants	polymyxin B
cyclophosphamide	probenecid
gold salts	proguanil
indomethacin	pyrazolone derivatives
kanamycin	sulfonamides
mandelic acid derivatives	sulfones
mefenamic acid	suramin
mephenesin	thiazides
mersalyl theophylline	viomycin
methenamine	

Normal range   *Adults:* Normally, a few red blood cells may be seen in the high power field. In the female, blood due to menstrual flow may be found. A catheterized specimen may contain blood because of urethral bleeding from the trauma caused by inserting the catheter. *Children:* Same as the range for adults.

Calcium Test (Sulkowitch)

This test measures roughly the amount of calcium in the urine. In hypoparathyroidism the urinary excretion of calcium is decreased. This test is therefore useful in cases of tetany to determine quickly whether the cause is hypoparathyroidism.

Food and drink restrictions   None.

Procedure for collecting specimen   A urine sample is placed in a bottle and sent to the laboratory.

Laboratory procedure   To a sample of urine is added an equal volume of Sulkowitch reagent. The extent of precipitation indicates roughly the amount of calcium. Absence of a precipitate suggests an abnormally low serum calcium.

Possible interfering materials and conditions   The urine calcium levels may be spuriously elevated if the patient has received any of the following:

> cholestyramine resin
> dihydrotachysterol
> nandrolone
> parathyroid injection
> vitamin D

There may be interference with the test if the patient has received thiazides or viomycin.

Normal range   *Adults:* A fine white precipitate indicates a normal concentration of serum calcium. *Children:* Same as the range for adults.

Catecholamines

This is a test for the presence of pheochromocytoma, a rare tumor of the chromaffin cells of the adrenal medulla and other parts of the sympathetic nervous system. Catecholamines are substances with chemical structures similar to those of epinephrine (Adrenalin) and norepinephrine (arterenol). When produced in the body, some of the unchanged material and some of the breakdown products containing the basic catecholamine structure are excreted in the urine. In cases of pheochromocytoma, the urinary levels of catecholamines are usually 3 to 100 times greater than normal. A correct diagnosis is usually life-saving, since pheochromocytomas produce severe hypertension, which is cured when the pheochromocytoma is removed surgically. In some psychiatric patients, catecholamine levels in the urine are slightly higher than normal, but not enough to be confused with pheochromocytoma. On the other hand, in the future, the slight catecholamine level elevations in psychiatric disorders may prove of considerable clinical and research value.

Food and drink restrictions   The patient should avoid coffee and bananas for 3 days.

Procedure for collecting specimen   The patient should take no drugs for 3 days before the beginning of the test. Notify the laboratory that the test has been ordered.

There are variations between laboratories in the use of a preservative. Some laboratories require a refrigerated specimen with no acid added, while others require the use of an acid preservative. For the latter, place 10 ml of concentrated hydrocholoric acid in a large bottle for a 24-hour urine specimen. Observe precautions to avoid spattering any of the acid on persons or materials. If possible, obtain a prepared bottle from the laboratory. Make sure there is no acid on the outside. Cap the bottle and place in the refrigerator. Use ordinary clean urine bottles to collect each urine specimen voided by the patient in a 24-hour period. As soon as each specimen is voided, pour it carefully into the large refrigerated bottle, and replace the latter in the refrigerator.

Laboratory procedure   The procedure for measuring catecholamines is so complicated that relatively few hospital laboratories perform it themselves. Instead, they send the samples to specialized laboratories. This means that the reporting of results is delayed. The basic method used is column chromatography, oxidation, and then photofluorometry.

Possible interfering materials and conditions   The urine catecholamine levels may be spuriously elevated by bananas and coffee, and also by many drugs. These drugs, listed by generic (official) name, include:

demethylchlortetracycline   quinine
epinephrine by inhalation   riboflavin (large doses)
hydralazine   salicylates (see Table 27)
methenamine   tetracyclines
methyldopa   vitamine B complex (large
nicotinic acid (large doses)   doses)
quinidine

Severe anxiety or anger may produce elevations of catecholamine levels.

Normal range *Adults:* Depending on the laboratory, this may
be 0 to 100 or 0 to 200 micrograms excreted in 24 hours. *Children:*
This test is not commonly performed on children. The normal range
for children is probably less than the normal range for adults because
of weight differences.

Chlorides, Quantitative

This examination is performed to evaluate the urinary excretion of
chlorides. It is useful in the management of cardiac patients on low
salt diets and in adjusting fluid and ion balance in postoperative cases.

Food and drink restrictions   None.

Procedure for collecting specimen   The total urine excreted over
a 24-hour period is collected in a large bottle.

Laboratory procedure   A simplified test, using a manufactured
tablet, is now replacing the more complex analytical chemical
techniques.

Possible interfering materials and conditions   There may be a
spurious elevation of urine chloride levels if the patient has taken
bromides.

Normal range   *Adults:* This may vary considerably with salt
intake and with perspiration. In general, most of the ingested
chloride, less that lost in perspiration, is excreted in the urine. Thus
there is really no "normal" or "abnormal" range and the values
obtained in this test are significant only in relation to the balance
between intake and output. Usually there are about 9 gm of sodium
chloride per liter of urine. *Children:* This test is not commonly
performed on children.

Concentration and Dilution

These tests measure the ability of the kidneys to concentrate and dilute urine, an indication of their functional capacity. Inadequate concentration or dilution of urine indicates some disorder of the tubules of the kidneys.

Procedure for collecting specimen   The procedures vary in different institutions. A fairly common one is the following:

First night

1. At supper the patient is restricted to 1 glass of fluid.
2. Thereafter, no food or drink is given until the end of the test.
3. The patient remains in bed as much as possible.
4. Before going to sleep the patient empties the bladder and the urine is discarded.
5. On wakening the patient passes a urine specimen, which is saved.
6. Second and third specimens are collected 1 and 2 hours later. The exact time of voiding each specimen is recorded.
7. After the third specimen the patient may have food and drink.

Second night

8. A regular supper is eaten.
9. No food or drink allowed thereafter, except as specified.
10. The patient is kept in bed as much as possible.
11. On wakening in the morning, the patient empties the bladder and the urine specimen is discarded.
12. After urination the patient is given 5 glasses of fluid to drink within 45 minutes. The fluid may be water, lemonade, or weak tea.
13. Urine is collected 1, 2, 3, and 4 hours after the patient has started drinking.
14. After the 4-hour specimen has been collected, the patient may have food and drink.

Laboratory procedure   The specific gravity of each urine specimen is measured with a urinometer.

Possible interfering materials and conditions   None reported yet.

Normal range *Adults:* For the concentration phase of the test, normal specific gravity is 1.025 or more; osmolality is 850 mOsm/L or more. For the dilution phase, normal specific gravity is about 1.003 to 1.005 in first urine specimen, and gradually increases thereafter. *Children:* Similar to that for adults.

Corticosteroids *See* 17 Hydroxy Corticosteroids

Creatinine

This is a test of kidney function and, at times, a check on the completeness of urinary collection. Creatinine is formed from creatine and is relatively constant from day to day in any individual. In cases of kidney impairment, urinary creatinine measurement, usually as part of the creatinine clearance test (p. 146), can help diagnose kidney failure. Sometimes, creatinine levels of 24-hour urine specimens are used to determine whether the collection was complete. However, the accuracy of this method of checking is open to question.

Food and drink restrictions Beginning at least 6 hours before the collection, and continuing throughout the collection, the patient should not receive large amounts of meat, poultry, fish, coffee, or tea.

Procedure for collecting specimen The patient empties his bladder completely and the urine is discarded. All urine passed during the next 24 hours, including a sample passed exactly 24 hours later, is collected without any preservative and stored in a refrigerator. Some hospitals use a collection period of less than 24 hours.

Laboratory procedure A colorimetric procedure is used.

Possible interfering materials and conditions Large amounts of meat, poultry, or fish could give spuriously high levels. Diuretic drugs may affect the results, but this is not certain.

Normal range *Adults:* This depends largely on muscle mass. Therefore, men have higher excretion levels than women and muscular individuals have higher excretion levels than the less muscular. At a major laboratory, the normal range is 21 to 26 mg/kg/24 hr for men, and 16 to 22 mg/kg/24 hr for women. *Children:* This test is not commonly performed on children because of problems in collection. The ranges would be lower in proportion to the lesser muscle mass.

Creatinine Clearance

This is a test of kidney glomerular function. When the serum creatinine level is in the normal range, 0.6 to 1.3 mg per 100 ml, the urinary excretion of creatinine depends almost entirely on the glomeruli. However, if serum creatinine levels rise above normal, the tubules excrete significant amounts of it, so that interpretation of creatinine clearance becomes complex. The creatinine clearance test is useful in two basic situations. It can be an early sign of glomerular damage and can produce abnormal results when the serum creatinine levels are still within normal limits. Also, it can be used to follow the course of known glomerular disease and to evaluate the effects of treatment.

Food and drink restrictions   Beginning at least 6 hours before the test and continuing throughout the test, the patient should not receive any meat, poultry, fish, tea, or coffee. Otherwise, he may have ordinary hospital foods. His water intake should be at least 100 ml/hr for the test period.

Procedure for collecting specimen
1. Urine: On the morning of the test, the patient empties his bladder completely, and the exact time is noted. This urine sample is discarded. The patient drinks a glass of water, and continues to drink water at a rate of at least 100 ml/hr. *All* urine passed during the next 24 hours is collected without any preservative, but is stored in a refrigerator. The exact time of the last voiding is also noted. Some laboratories use a collection period of less than 24 hours.

2. Blood: On the morning of the test 5 ml of *venous* blood is collected in a collecting tube with a red stopper.

Laboratory procedure   The serum creatinine level is measured as described under creatinine, as well as the amount of creatinine in the 24-hour urine specimen. From these measurements, the volume of serum cleared of creatinine per minute is calculated.

Possible interfering materials and conditions   Foods with high creatinine content (meat, poultry, fish) may interfere with the results. Coffee and tea may interfere because of their diuretic effects. Strenuous exercise may also interfere. Diuretic drugs may give spurious results, and should not be given for at least a day before the test or during the test.

Normal range *Adults:* The normal creatinine clearance is 100 to 140 ml/min. *Children:* This test is not usually performed on children.

Culture *See* Urine Culture, Chapter 2

Delta Aminolevulinic Acid *See* Aminolevulinic Acid (Urine)

Diacetic (Aceto-Acetic) Acid *See* Ketone Bodies

d-Xylose Tolerance Test (oral) *See* Xylose

E 3 *See* Estriol (Urine)

Estriol

The measurement of the level of this hormone in the urine is often an aid in diagnosing fetal distress during pregnancy. When serious fetal distress occurs, the maternal urinary estriol levels tend to fall. The normal levels vary considerably among individuals. Furthermore, the levels change as pregnancy progresses. Accordingly, a more complex than usual method of determining abnormality is employed. Successive measurements of estriol levels are made. If there is a decrease of at least 40% on two successive days, or a decrease of 20% in the average of two successive weeks, one may presume that there is some fetal distress.

Food and drink restrictions None.

Procedure for collecting specimen Place 15 ml of concentrated HCl in a urine collection bottle. Then, collect a 24-hour specimen and send to the laboratory.

Laboratory procedure A commonly used procedure involves gas chromatographic analysis of the specimen.

Possible interfering materials and conditions None reported yet.

Normal range After the 35th week of pregnancy, the level is usually 20 mg/24 hr or higher.

Fermentation Test for Sugar

This test is no longer in common use.

Friedman Test

This test for pregnancy, using a female rabbit, is no longer in common use.

Frog Test for Pregnancy

This test is no longer in common use.

Glucose   *See* Sugar

Glucose Tolerance   *See* Glucose Tolerance, Chapter 3

Gravindex   *See* Immunologic Test for Pregnancy

Hemostix   *See* Blood, Urine, page 139

Heroin   *See* Morphine

5-HIAA   *See* 5-Hydroxyindoleacetic Acid

Hogben

This is another test for pregnancy, using a South African toad. It is no longer in common use.

Homogentisic Acid

This is a test for alkaptonuria, a rather rare metabolic disease. In this condition, the oxidation of tyrosine does not proceed fully along the normal pathways, and an intermediary metabolite, homogentisic acid, is excreted in the urine. The urine is normally colored when voided, but turns dark on standing. Furthermore, pigment is deposited in the eye, ear, nose, and tendons of the hand. One or more of these signs may bring the patient to medical attention. Alkaptonuria is not a particularly dangerous condition. Its major disadvantage is that it is associated with the development of arthritis in later life. There is no specific treatment available at this time. An accurate diagnosis of alkaptonuria is of great benefit to the patient and his family, however, since it should relieve any concern that a fatal or life-shortening disorder may be present.

Food and drink restrictions   None.

Procedure for collecting specimen   Ordinarily, any fresh urine sample may be used for this test.

Laboratory procedure   Several procedures are available. The simplest is the addition of alkali, which turns the urine black. Homogentisic acid will also give a positive reaction to the Benedict reagent in a common test for sugar.

Possible interfering materials and conditions   The level of homogentisic acid may seem falsely elevated if the patient has received salicylates (Table 27) in the preceding 3 days.

Normal range   Normally there is no homogentisic acid in the urine. Salicylates may produce milligram quantities of gentisic acid, a similar material. However, in alkaptonuria, much larger amounts of homogentisic acid are found.

5-Hydroxyindoleacetic Acid (5-HIAA)

This is a test for the presence of a carcinoid tumor. These rare tumors are found mainly in the appendix, but occasionally in the small or large intestine. The cells of the carcinoid tumor secrete serotinin, which is broken down to 5-hydroxyindoleacetic acid, producing a marked elevation in the usual urinary levels of this material. Carcinoid tumors have a low degree of malignancy, so that reasonably prompt removal gives a high chance of complete cure. Recently, it was found that in a few rare cases, noncarcinoid tumors may also produce high urinary levels of 5-HIAA.

Food and drink restrictions   The patient must not eat any bananas for at least 3 days before the test.

Procedure for collecting specimen   The patient must be kept off most drugs for at least 3 full days before starting the collection of urine. The total urine for a 24-hour period is collected and sent to the laboratory. The specimen should be kept refrigerated.

Laboratory procedure   The laboratory may do a screening test first, and then if that is positive do a quantitative measurement. Some laboratories will do the quantitative measurement directly. The quantitative measurement is done with a spectrophotometer.

Possible interfering materials and conditions   There may be an elevated urinary excretion of 5-hydroxyindoleacetic acid in patients with nontropical sprue, but this elevation is generally much less than that found in cases of carcinoid tumor.

The urine 5-HIAA levels may be increased if the patient has, in the preceding 3 days, eaten bananas, plantains, or certain other fruits not yet identified. The following drugs, listed by official (generic) name, may also produce increased levels if taken in the preceding 3 days:

acetanilid	methysergide maleate
glyceryl guaiacolate	phenothiazines
mephenesin	reserpine
methocarbamol	

The urinary 5-HIAA levels may be artifically depressed if the patient has received one of the phenothiazine-type drugs (see Table 25).

Normal range   *Adults:* For screening test: Normally there is no 5-HIAA in the urine. For quantitative measurement: 2 to 10 mg in 24 hours. *Children:* This test is not ordinarily performed on children, but presumably the normal range should be similar to that for adults.

17 Hydroxy Corticosteroids   (Also known as 17 Hydroxy-steroids, abbreviated as 17-OHCS)

This is primarily a test of adrenal cortex function. The adrenal cortex produces corticosteroids that are altered and then excreted largely in the urine. The level of 17 hydroxy corticosteroids may, therefore, give an indication of the rate at which the adrenals are producing the corticosteroids. In cases of hyperadrenalism (Cushing's syndrome) the urinary levels are higher than normal. However, the reverse is not necessarily true. In cases of hypoadrenalism, the urinary levels of 17 hydroxy corticosteroids may be within the normal range. If adrenal cortical underfunction is suspected but the urinary levels of 17-OHCS are normal, the physician may administer ACTH and retest the urinary 17-OHCS excretion. If adrenal cortical function is normal, the urinary excretion of 17-OHCS will rise markedly after ACTH. However, if adrenal cortical function is poor, the urinary levels of 17-OHCS will not rise much.

Food and drink restrictions None.

Procedure for collecting specimen Place a large, clean urine collection container in the refrigerator. Collect each urine sample from the patient during a 24-hour period in a regular clean urine bottle and pour it into the large refrigerated container. During the 24-hour collection period, the patient should drink 6 to 8 glasses of fluids.

Laboratory procedure A spectrophotometric method is used.

Possible interfering materials and conditions Many drugs interfere with this test, and it is advisable to avoid administering any medications to the patient for at least 3 days before the test. It is of some interest to note that while cortisone and several of its derivatives tend to elevate the urinary levels of 17-OHCS, some of the high-potency derivatives, such as dexamethasone, tend to decrease the urinary levels. Apparently, the reason for this effect of dexamethasone is that by inhibiting ACTH production, it causes a diminution of adrenal cortical secretion, while its own breakdown products are low in quantity because of low dosage. Some of the substances known to interfere with this measurement are the following, listed by official (generic) name:

acetazolamide	digoxin
chloral hydrate	estrogens
chlordiazepoxide	ethinamate
chlormerodrin	glutethimide
chlorothiazide	hydralazine
chlorpromazine	hydroxyzine
colchicine	iodides
corticosteroids	meprobamate
cortisone	oleandomycin
dexamethasone	oral contraceptives
dextroamphetamine	paraldehyde
digitoxin	penicillin

perphenazine	quinidine
phenazopyridine	quinine
phenothiazines	reserpine
piperidine	spironolactone
prochlorperazine	testosterone
promazine	triacetyloleandomycin

Normal range *Adults:* 4 to 14 mg in 24 hours. *Children:* Lower than the range for adults, but specific value ranges for various ages are not available.

Immunologic Test for Pregnancy

This test appears to be highly accurate. It has advantages over the older pregnancy tests such as Aschheim-Zondek, Friedman, and Hogben in that it does not require the use of live animals and that a result is obtained in a shorter time. The immunologic test is sensitive enough to be positive in most cases of pregnancy by the 13th day after the first missed period (41 days after the onset of the last menstrual period). Since the test is based on the presence of chorionic gonadotropin in the urine, it will also be positive in cases of chorionepithelioma and hydatidiform mole.

Food and drink restrictions None.

Procedure for collecting specimen Any urine specimen may be used provided it is not grossly contaminated and does not contain blood. However, more concentrated specimens (specific gravity over 1.015) provide more accurate results.

Laboratory procedure A drop of urine is placed on a slide, a drop of antiserum to chorionic gonadotropin added, and the two are mixed well for 30 seconds. Then, 2 drops of prepared antigen (latex particles coated with human chorionic gonadotropin) are added and mixed gently. If agglutination of the latex particles occurs within 2 minutes, the test is negative. If there is no agglutination within 2 minutes, the test is positive.

Possible interfering materials and conditions Chorionepithelioma and hydatidiform mole may produce positive test results.

Normal range In the absence of pregnancy, the reaction is negative.

Ketone Bodies, Urine

This test is helpful in diagnosing ketosis, a type of acidosis produced by faulty metabolism. In improperly or uncontrolled diabetes, sugar is not utilized properly, and excessive fat is metabolized. The fats produce ketone bodies, betahydroxybutyric acid, acetoacetic (diacetic) acid, and acetone. When the levels of these compounds in the blood rise, some of the compounds spill over into the urine.

There may also be ketone bodies in the urine in starvation and in other major metabolic disturbances. This test is replacing the older individual tests for acetone and acetoacetic (diacetic) acid in the urine.

Food and drink restrictions   None.

Procedure for collecting specimen   A urine sample is placed in a bottle and sent to the laboratory.

Laboratory procedure   Several procedures are available, including commercial packages containing tablet and paper strip (Ketostix).

Possible interfering materials   This will depend on the laboratory procedure used. Preparations of levodopa (L-Dopa, Larodopa, Levodopa) may, under certain circumstances, give false positive reactions.

Normal range   *Adults:* Normally, no ketone bodies are present in urine. *Children:* Same as for adults.

17 K   *See* 17-Ketosteroid Excretion and 17-Ketogenic Steroids

17-Ketogenic Steroids

This test is a sensitive measurement of adrenocortical function. In some rare cases of Cushing's disease and adrenogenital syndrome, the 17-hydroxycorticosteroid levels may be normal but the 17-ketogenic steroid levels will be elevated. The levels are also elevated in adrenal carcinoma, ACTH therapy, and severe stress. Levels are decreased in Addison's disease and panhypopituitarism, at the ending of corticosteroid therapy, and in general wasting.

Food and drink restrictions   None.

Procedure for collecting specimen   A 24-hour urine specimen is needed. The collecting bottle should be kept refrigerated.

Laboratory procedure   A complicated method is used, with final colorimetric determination.

Possible interfering materials and conditions   The 17-ketogenic steroid level may be elevated if the patient has taken one of the following drugs, listed by official (generic) name:

chlordiazepoxide   penicillin
cortisone   phenothiazines (Table 25)
ethinamate   spironolactone
meprobamate (Table 23)   triacetyloleandomycin
oleandomycin

The 17-ketogenic steroid level may be decreased if the patient has received any of the following:

chlorothiazide   piperidine
cortisone derivatives of quinidine
   high potency   quinine
methyprylon   secobarbital
paraldehyde   thiazides
phenazopyridine

Many drugs may interfere with the test procedure and make an accurate reading impossible. Such drugs include those listed above plus the following:

betamethasone   oral contraceptives
dexamethasone   probenecid
estrogens   pyrazinamide

Normal range

Adults: Men: 5 to 20 mg/24 hr
            Women: 3 to 15 mg/24 hr

Children (male and female):   2 to 5 years: less than
                                   2 mg/24 hr
                                5 to 10 years: 3 to 6 mg/24 hr
                                10 years to adulthood: rising to
                                   adult levels

17-Ketosteroid Excretion

The 17-ketosteroids are male hormones with a ketone group on the 17th carbon atom of the phenanthrene ring. In men, two-thirds of these hormones are produced by the adrenals and only one-third by the testes. In women, virtually all of these materials are secreted by the adrenals. Accordingly, it should be clear that, although they are male hormones, the level of 17-ketosteroid excretion is usually more important in diagnosing disorders of the adrenals than disorders of the testes.

In children, the level of 17-ketosteroids is normally very low. Low levels of these compounds are found in adrenal hypofunction from any cause, including Addison's disease, myxedema, pituitary hypofunction, and many types of severe debilitating illness.

High levels of 17-ketosteroids are found in certain types of adrenal or testicular hyperfunction. In women with virilizing syndromes, the 17-ketosteroid excretion is usually moderately elevated.

Very marked elevations, over 100 mg/day, suggest either carcinoma of the adrenal cortex or the extremely rare interstitial cell tumor of the testis.

Food and drink restrictions None.

Procedure for collecting specimen This varies from laboratory to laboratory. Some require only refrigeration of the urine. Others require acidification in addition to refrigeration.

Into a large bottle, usually of gallon size, 3 ml of acetic acid is placed as a preservative. The patient's urine for a 24-hour period is then collected in this bottle. If the patient has been receiving bicarbonate of soda, a greater amount of acetic acid might be required to maintain the acidity of the specimen. The collection bottle should be kept refrigerated.

Laboratory procedure A colorimetric test is commonly used.

Possible interfering materials and conditions The 17-ketosteroid level may be elevated if the patient has taken one of the following drugs, listed by official (generic) name:

chlordiazepoxide   ethinamate
cortisone   meprobamate (Table 23)

oleandomycin   spironolactone
penicillin   triacetyloleandomycin
phenothiazines (Table 25)

The 17-ketosteroid level may be decreased if the patient has received any of the following:

chlorothiazide   piperidine
cortisone derivatives of quinidine
   high potency   quinine
methylprylon   secobarbital
paraldehyde   thiazides
phenazopyridine

The test procedure may be interfered with by many drugs, making an accurate reading impossible. Such drugs include those listed above plus the following:

betamethasone   oral contraceptives
dexamethasone   probenecid
estrogens   pyrazinamide

Normal range

Adults: Men: 8 to 20 mg/day
            Women: 5 to 15 mg/day

Children: under 1 year: less than 1 mg/day
              1 to 4 years: less than 2 mg/day
              5 to 8 years: less than 3 mg/day
              9 to 12 years: about 3 mg/day
              13 to 16 years: rises gradually to the normal range
                 for adults

Lead

In suspected lead poisoning the determination of lead concentration in the urine may aid in diagnosis.

Food and drink restrictions   The patient must be on a low calcium diet for at least 3 days before the test to mobilize the lead from the bones.

Procedure for collecting specimen   Collect a 24-hour specimen in a special large bottle.

Laboratory procedure   Spectrographic methods are preferred.

Possible interfering materials and conditions   None reported yet.

Normal range   *Adults:* Less than 100 mcg/24 hrs. *Children:* Same as that for adults.

Melanin

This test is an aid in the diagnosis of melanoma. Melanin or its precursor, melanogen, appears in the urine in this disease but is also found in several other conditions. Melanin colors the urine brown or black. Melanogen is colorless.

Food and drink restrictions   None.

Procedure for collecting specimen   A urine sample is placed in a bottle and sent to the laboratory.

Laboratory procedure   Sodium nitroprusside and sodium hydroxide are added to a sample of urine. If a deep red color appears, glacial acetic acid is added and the instantaneous production of a blue color indicates melanogen.

Possible interfering materials and conditions   None reported yet.

Normal range   Normally there is no melanin or melanogen in the urine.

Melanogen   *See* Melanin

Microscopic Tests

Microscopic examination of the urinary sediment may reveal important information about the condition of the urinary tract. Red blood cells in males, or in females who are not of menstrual age, suggest bleeding somewhere along the tract, from glomerulus to urethra. When red blood cells are found, further studies are usually performed to determine the exact source of the blood.

Many white blood cells (leukocytes) in specimens from males, or in clean-catch specimens from females, suggest infection of the urinary tract.

Casts in the urine suggest some disorder of the kidney tubules.

Crystals of certain kinds (sulfonamide, for example) may indicate a need for change in therapeutic regimen.

Food and drink restrictions   None.

Procedure for collecting specimen   A urine specimen is placed in a bottle and sent to the laboratory.

Laboratory procedure   A sample of the urine is centrifuged and the sediment examined microscopically.

Possible interfering materials and conditions   None reported yet.

Normal range   Laboratories vary in their interpretation of normal range. Some experts consider that 2 or 3 red blood cells per high power field is normal for males. Others consider 1 to 2 red cells per high power field the upper limit of normal. To some extent, this depends on how many fields are counted. A few white blood cells (leukocytes) per high power field is also normal for males. In urine of females of menstrual age, substantial quantities of both red and white blood cells may be found. A few casts may be present normally, but large numbers of casts suggest kidney disease.

Morphine

This test is performed to determine whether the patient has taken morphine or heroin during the preceding 24 hours. (Heroin is metabolized to morphine in the body.) Its usual use is in methadone maintenance programs for heroin addicts, to see if the patient is abstaining from heroin. The test for urine morphine is positive only if the patient has taken morphine or heroin within the previous 24 hours. Hardcore heroin addicts who are being treated by methadone maintenance are, for months or years, completely unreliable and untrustworthy, and therefore objective tests are needed to monitor their progress.

Food and drink restrictions   None.

Procedure for collecting specimen   The urine specimen must be collected under the direct observation of a member of the clinic or hospital staff who actually sees the patient urinate into the container and who then takes the container from the patient. Under no circumstances can the patient be trusted when he states that a sample is his, or that it was passed at a particular time.

If a urine sample is collected daily (7 times a week), one can be sure of the validity of the results. However, if a urine sample is collected and analyzed less frequently, there must be a completely randomized and unpredictable pattern of collection days, so that when the patient arrives at the clinic, he does not know whether a urine sample will be required or not. If a clinic requires a urine test only 5 days a week, some patients may revert to heroin on Friday evening and Saturday, confident that their urine specimens from Monday through Friday will be negative. If a clinic has a randomized collection program, it should be arranged so that Saturdays and Sundays are included in the pattern.

No special preservatives are needed for the urine.

Laboratory procedure   The morphine is identified by thin layer chromatography.

Possible interfering materials and conditions   None reported yet.

Normal range   Normally, there is no morphine in the urine.

Myoglobin

Myoglobin is a normal constituent of muscle, similar in some respects to hemoglobin. In some conditions in which severe muscle destruction occurs, the myoglobin leaks out of the muscle, into the blood, and thence to the urine. It is quite soluble in an alkaline urine, but if the urine is acid, the myoglobin may precipitate in the kidney tubules, blocking them and causing kidney damage. In severe cases, the kidney damage can be fatal. The most striking example is the so-called crush syndrome, in which large muscle masses (usually the thigh) are crushed in an accident, and myoglobin appears in the urine. Myoglobinuria in lesser degree also occurs in dermatomyositis, after eating fish that have been poisoned by factory wastes, and in other conditions of muscle destruction. Myoglobin colors the urine brown or red.

Food and drink restrictions   None.

Procedure for collecting specimen   A urine sample is placed in a bottle and sent to the laboratory.

Laboratory procedure   A positive hemastix test of the urine indicates the presence of either hemoglobin or myoglobin.

Possible interfering materials and conditions None reported yet.

Normal range Normally, no myoglobin is found in the urine in quantities sufficient to give a positive reaction by this method.

Myoglobin, Quantitative

This is a test for myocardial infarction. Within 24 hours after an infarction, the necrotic heart muscle releases myoglobin into the serum, and from there it is excreted in the urine. If a urine sample, diluted 4 or 8 times, still shows myoglobin, there is a strong likelihood of myocardial infarction. The test is only valuable within 24 hours or so after the infarction.

Food and drink restrictions None.

Procedure for collecting specimen A fresh urine specimen is sent to the laboratory.

Laboratory procedure A specific antiserum is tested against serial dilutions of the urine.

Possible interfering materials and conditions These include any conditions resulting in major muscle destruction and paroxysmal myoglobinuria. Examples are: excessive, unusual exercise; beating; bullet wounds; crush injury; acute dermatomyositis and polymyositis; fish poisoning; and sea snake bite. Fortunately, these conditions are rarely present in the patient suspected of having a myocardial infarction.

Normal range *Adults:* Normally there is no myoglobin in the urine. *Children:* This test is not performed on children.

17-OH *See* 17 Hydroxy Corticosteroids

17-OHCS *See* 17 Hydroxy Corticosteroids

pH

This is a measure of the degree of acidity or alkalinity of the urine. The kidney maintains the blood at the correct pH by excreting into the urine any excess ions that might alter the pH of the blood. The urinary pH, therefore, varies widely and changes do not indicate abnormality. However, in certain situations it is advisable to have an acid or alkaline urine, and the pH measurement is important. When sulfadiazine is administered or when there is marked hemolysis or destruction of muscle tissue (crush syndrome), an alkaline urine is needed to keep the excreted substances soluble. Sulfadiazine and the products of hemolysis and muscle destruction are quite soluble in an alkaline urine, but in acid urine they precipitate and may cause urinary blockage and death. In treatment with certain urinary tract antiseptics (methenamine) an acid urine is needed. In bladder infections the urine may be highly alkaline because bacteria transform urea into ammonia.

Food and drink restrictions   None.

Procedure for collecting specimen   A urine specimen is placed in a bottle and sent to the laboratory. The urinary pH is important in infants being treated with sulfadiazine, but collection of a urine sample may be difficult. A simple expedient is to place a strip of testing paper inside the diaper at each change. The pH of the urine is then determined by the color of the paper. Urine pH tends to change as soon as bacterial contamination from air or other sources occurs. Therefore, the pH should be measured promptly.

Laboratory procedure   Usually a test with a strip of indicator paper is adequate. Sometimes a pH meter is used.

Possible interfering materials and conditions   None reported yet.

Normal range   *Adults:* pH 4.8 to 8.0. *Children:* Same as the range for adults.

Phenolsulfonphthalein (PSP) Test

This is a test of the ability of the kidney tubules to excrete a dye. The urinary excretion of injected phenolsulfonphthalein is decreased in chronic nephritis and urinary tract obstructions. It may be increased in certain liver diseases.

Food and drink restrictions   None.

Procedure for collecting specimen   It is not necessary for the patient to empty the bladder before the test is begun. The patient drinks two glasses of water. Thirty minutes later, the physician injects 1 ml of phenolsulfonphthalein intravenously, taking 3 minutes for the injection. The exact time of injection is noted.

Urine specimens are then collected in separate containers at intervals of 15, 30, 60, and 120 minutes after injection of the dye and sent to the laboratory.

Laboratory procedure   The urine samples are alkalinized to bring out the maximum color and compared to standards in a colorimeter.

Possible interfering materials and conditions   In liver disease, there may be a spurious increase in phenolsulfonphalein excretion.

In multiple myeloma and hypoalbuminemia, there may be a spurious decrease in phenolsulfonphthalein excretion.

The PSP levels may be elevated by several drugs. Those currently known, listed by official (generic) name, include:

anthraquinone derivatives   phenolphthalein
cascara   probenecid
danthron   pyridium
ethoxazene   radiographic contrast
novobiocin   media
phenazopyridine drugs   rhubarb extracts
    (see Table 17)

The PSP readings may be decreased by the following:

diuretics
penicillin
salicylates (see Table 27)
sulfonamides

Normal range   *Adults:* The most sensitive part of the test is the first 15 minutes, during which period from 10% to 50% of the dye should be excreted. *Children:* This test is not commonly performed on children.

Phenylketonuria Test

This test is designed to uncover early cases of phenylketonuria (phenylpyruvic oligophrenia). In this condition the patient—an infant—is unable to properly metabolize phenylalanine, an essential amino acid. As a result, pathologic metabolic end products are formed which lead to permanent mental deficiency. If the disorder is recognized early, a phenylalanine deficient diet can be given and the mental deficiency avoided. Accordingly, it is important to recognize the disorder as soon as possible. In some hospitals a routine diaper test is performed on all infants over 4 weeks of age, since infants with this disorder excrete phenylpyruvic acid in the urine after the age of 3 weeks.

In many states, the law requires that every infant be tested for phenylketonuria between the fourth and tenth weeks of life. At least two urine tests, a week apart, are required. Positive results must be reported to the Board of Health.

A blood test (see p. 71) is useful at ages as low as three days, so that it is being used instead of the urine test in many hospital laboratories.

Food and drink restrictions   None.

Procedure for collecting specimen   Several pieces of absorbent or filter paper are placed in the baby's diaper by the mother or nurse. After they have been wet with urine, they are dried and sent to the laboratory.

Laboratory procedure   A dried paper strip is tested with a drop of 10% ferric chloride solution. If phenylpyruvic acid is present the paper turns green, and the green color fades in 5 minutes. If the reaction is positive or doubtful, more precise chemical tests can be performed on the other papers for confirmation.

Possible interfering materials and conditions   The phenylketonuria test may be interfered with if the patient has received chlorpromazine, aspirin, or other salicylates (Table 27), since ferric chloride produces a pink color with metabolites of these drugs.

Normal range   *Adults:* This test is not commonly performed on adults. *Children:* Normally there is no phenylpyruvic acid in the urine.

Porphobilinogen

Porphobilinogen is a precursor of the porphyrins. Large amounts are excreted in acute intermittent porphyria, in some cases of hepatitis, and in disseminated cancer. The test is done primarily to help diagnose acute intermittent porphyria. In that condition, there are attacks of colicky abdominal pain. Porphobilinogen is almost always excreted during an attack. It may or may not be excreted between attacks.

Food and drink restrictions None.

Procedure for collecting specimen A fresh urine specimen should be collected during or immediately after an attack of colicky abdominal pain. It should be protected from light. A qualitative test may be done on 20 ml or more of any urine specimen. A quantitative test requires a 24-hour specimen, which must be refrigerated and protected from light. Some laboratories also require that 5 gm of anhydrous sodium carbonate be placed in the 24-hour collecting bottle to maintain an alkaline pH.

Laboratory procedure For qualitative screening tests, a paper indicating strip is used. For quantitative measurements, a colorimetric method is used.

Possible interfering materials and conditions Sulfonamides, procaine, and other, unidentified materials are reported to interfere with this test. Until more exact information becomes available, it would be wise to assume that any of the drugs that interfere with measurement of porphyrin levels in the urine (*see* Porphyrins) may also interfere with measurement of porphobilinogen levels.

Normal range *Adults:* Qualitative screening: Normally there is no porphobilinogen in the urine. Quantitative: 2 mg/24 hr. *Children:* Similar to the range for adults.

Porphyrins

Porphyrins are pigments, similar to bilirubin, and probably come from the hemoglobin of the blood. Normally there is an insignificant amount of porphyrins in the urine. In certain conditions, such as toxic liver damage, lead poisoning, some blood disorders, pellagra, and congenital porphyria, the urinary excretion of porphyrins rises.

Food and drink restrictions None.

Procedure for collecting specimen The total urine excreted by the patient over a 24-hour period is collected in a large bottle. The sample should be kept refrigerated and protected from light.

Laboratory procedure A spectroscopic procedure is used.

Possible interfering materials and conditions The urine porphyrin level may be increased if the patient has received one of a number of drugs. The list, by official (generic) name, includes:

acriflavine	penicillin
alcohol	phenazopyridine
antipyretics	phenothiazines (see
barbiturates (see Table 18)	Table 25)
chloroquine	phenylhydrazine
chlorpromazine	procaine
ethoxazene	sedatives and hypnotics
oxytetracycline	sulfonamides

Normal range   *Adults:* A minute quantity may normally be found in the urine. *Children:* Same as the range for adults.

Protein   *See* Albumin

PSP   *See* Phenolsulfonphthalein Test

Slide Test for Pregnancy   *See* Immunologic Test for Pregnancy

Specific Gravity

This measurement indicates the degree of concentration of dissolved material in the urine. Ordinarily the specific gravity rises when the fluid intake is low and falls when fluid intake is high. In certain kidney disorders involving the tubules the urine is not concentrated or diluted beyond relatively narrow limits.

Food and drink restrictions   None.

Procedure for collecting specimen   A urine sample is placed in a bottle and sent to the laboratory.

Laboratory procedure   The extent to which a standard urinometer sinks in the urine determines the specific gravity. A refractometer test is becoming more common, since it requires only a drop of urine.

Possible interfering materials and conditions   The specific gravity may be increased if the patient has received dextran or radiographic contrast media.

Normal range   *Adults:* 1.001 to 1.035. *Children:* Newborns tend to have a specific gravity close to 1.012. As they grow older, their urine specific gravity varies within the range for adults.

Sugar, Qualitative

In some disorders sugar is found in the urine. This occurs most often in diabetes mellitus, but it may also occur in other metabolic disorders of varying importance. Because of its simplicity this test is usually employed as a screening procedure to discover diabetes. If sugar is found, other tests may then be ordered to determine the type of sugar.

Food and drink restrictions None.

Procedure for collecting specimen A urine sample is placed in a bottle and sent to the laboratory.

Laboratory procedure The more complex tests of the past have now been replaced with simplified dip-stick tests and, in some cases, tablet tests. However, chemical tests may be used to confirm positive reactions in the simpler tests.

Possible interfering materials and conditions A large number of drugs may produce false positive reactions for sugar in the urine. Sometimes the type of test procedure used by the laboratory may make a difference. The drugs reported able to produce false positive, or spurious, elevations in urine sugar levels *in at least one type of test* include the following, listed by their official (generic) names:

acetanilid	isoniazid
aminosalicylic acid	metaxalone
antipyrine	nalidixic acid
ascorbic acid (large doses)	nicotinic acid
aspidium oleoresin	nitrofurantoin
bismuth salts	nitrofurazone
carinamide	para-aminosalicylic acid
cephalothin	penicillin
chloral hydrate	phenacetin
chloramphenicol	probenecid
chlortetracycline	pyrazolone derivatives
cinchophen	quinethazone
corticosteroids	salicylates (Table 27)
diatrizoate	streptomycin
edathamil	sulfonamides
ephedrine (large doses)	tetracyclines
ethacrynic acid	thiazides
gluconates	trioxazine
indomethacin	vaginal powders (some)

Normal range *Adults:* Normally, there is only a small amount of sugar in the urine, not enough to give a positive screening test. *Children:* Same as the range for adults.

Sugar, Quantitative

This test is performed on some diabetics to determine the extent of sugar loss.

Food and drink restrictions None.

Procedure for collecting specimen A 24-hour urine specimen is collected in a clean bottle and sent to the laboratory. The specimen should be kept refrigerated, and preserved with some fresh thymol or sodium fluoride.

Laboratory procedure A sample of the urine is titrated with Benedict's quantitative solution. The disappearance of color from the Benedict's solution marks the end point.

Possible interfering materials and conditions A large number of drugs may produce false positive reactions for sugar in the urine. Sometimes the type of test procedure used by the laboratory may make a difference. The drugs reported able to produce false positive, or spurious elevations in urine sugar levels, listed by official (generic) name, include:

acetanilid
aminosalicylic acid
antipyrine
ascorbic acid (large doses)
aspidium oleoresin
bismuth salts
carinamide
cephalothin
chloral hydrate
chloramphenicol
chlortetracycline
cinchophen
corticosteroids
diatrizoate
edathamil
ephedrine (large doses)
ethacrynic acid

gluconates
indomethacin
isoniazid
metaxalone
nalidixic acid
nicotinic acid
nitrofurantoin
nitrofurazone
para-aminosalicylic acid
penicillin
phenacetin
probenecid
pyrazolone derivatives
quinethazone
salicylates (Table 27)
streptomycin
sulfonamides

tetracyclines   trioxazine
thiazides   vaginal powders (some)

Normal range   *Adults:* 116 to 656 mg/24 hr (total sugar). *Children:* Similar to the range for adults.

Sulkowitch Test   *See* Calcium Test (Sulkowitch)

Urea Clearance

This test is seldom performed these days because it has been replaced by less cumbersome, more useful tests of kidney function.

Urobilinogen

This is a test to aid in the differential diagnosis between complete and incomplete obstruction of the biliary tract. Increases in urinary urobilinogen (a breakdown product of hemoglobin) occur in many conditions, including hemolytic diseases, liver damage, and severe infections. However, in complete obstructive jaundice without infection there is ordinarily no excess of urobilinogen in the urine.

When antibiotics are being administered, this test may not be accurate. Antibiotics inhibit growth of intestinal bacteria and therefore interfere with the production of urobilinogen in the intestine.

Food and drink restrictions   None.

Procedure for collecting specimen   Laboratories vary in their requirements. Some require only a single, fresh urine specimen. More commonly, a 2-hour specimen is needed. The sample is kept in a brown bottle, protected from light, and taken to the laboratory without delay.

Laboratory procedure   For semiquantitative screening, dipsticks are available. For quantitative measurements, a colorimetric procedure is used.

Possible interfering materials and conditions   The urobilinogen level may be falsely elevated if the patient has recently received any of the following materials:

amidopyrine (Pyramidon) Novocaine
antipyrine p-Aminosalicylic acid
bromsulphalein (BSP) phenazopyridine (Pyridium)
chlorpromazine (Thorazine) (see Table 17)
diatrizoate (Hypaque) Thoradex

Urobilinogen levels may be reduced if the patient has received an antibiotic or chemotherapeutic agent which affects the microorganisms in the intestine.

Normal range *Adults:* A maximum excretion rate of 2.5 mg in 24 hours, or not over 2 Ehrlich units in 2 hours. *Children:* This test is not commonly performed on children. Probably the normal range after one month is lower than the normal range for adults.

Vanilmandelic Acid (VMA)

This is a test for pheochromocytoma (see Catecholamines, p. 141). Pheochromocytoma is a rare tumor of the chromaffin cells of the adrenal medulla and other parts of the sympathetic nervous system. Such tumors secrete excessive amounts of catecholamines like epinephrine (adrenaline) and norepinephrine (arterenol). The metabolic breakdown of these catecholamines in the body results in several products, of which vanilmandelic acid (VMA) is the most prominent. Accordingly, the discovery of a high level of vanilmandelic acid in the urine may be an important aid to the diagnosis of pheochromocytoma.

Two related tumors, neuroblastoma and ganglioneuroblastoma, found mainly in infants and young children, also produce elevated urinary levels of vanilmandelic acid.

This is a rather nonspecific test, and may give false positive results unless closely correlated with clinical observations of the patient's signs and symptoms.

Food and drink restrictions Certain foods and beverages are believed capable of producing phenoxyacids in the urine, and these may give false reactions. Accordingly, such items must be omitted for at least 3 days before the test and during the collection of the urine.

At our present level of knowledge, the foods and beverages to be omitted are chocolate, coffee, tea, vanilla flavoring, and all fruits. It is likely that other dietary items will also be found to interfere with this test.

Procedure for collecting specimen   The patient should take no drugs for 3 days before the beginning of the test. Some laboratories require the use of acid as a preservative; others ask that no acid be used. Check policies of the laboratory involved. If acid is used, place 10 ml of *concentrated* hydrochloric acid in a large bottle for a 24-hour urine specimen. Observe precautions to avoid spattering any of the acid on persons or materials. If possible, obtain a prepared bottle from the laboratory. Make sure there is no acid on the outside. Place all urine voided during 24 hours in the large bottle. Whether or not acid is used, keep the specimen refrigerated during the 24-hour period.

Laboratory procedure   A spectrophotometric procedure is used.

Possible interfering materials and conditions   Many foods and drugs are known to interfere with vanilmandelic acid measurements, and others will probably be added to the list in the future. For this reason, all drugs should, if possible, be discontinued at least 3 days before the test and during the collection of the urine sample.

Foods and beverages that may give spuriously elevated urine vanilmandelic acid levels include:

> bananas
> chocolate
> coffee
> tea
> vanilla flavoring

Drugs that may give spuriously elevated urinary vanilmandelic acid levels include:

anileridine (Leritine)	methenamine (Mandelamine)
cough medicines (some)	methocarbamol (Robaxin)
glyceryl guaiacolate	salicylates (see Table 27)
mephenesin (Tolserol)	

In addition, reserpine derivatives (Table 26) may interfere with the reading of vanilmandelic acid levels.

Normal range   *Adults:* The normal amount of vanilmandelic acid in a 24-hour urine specimen is not more than 7.5 mg. *Children:*

This test is not commonly performed on children. Probably the normal range is no greater than the normal range for adults.

Vitamin C   *See* Ascorbic Acid

VMA   *See* Vanilmandelic Acid

d-Xylose Tolerance Test (Oral)

This test is less commonly used than it formerly was. It is a test of the ability of the gastrointestinal tract to absorb nutrients. Several disorders of absorption can be corrected by appropriate treatment if they are accurately diagnosed.

The d-xylose is ordinarily absorbed by the gastrointestinal tract and then excreted by the kidney. If, after ingestion, the amount found in the urine is low (assuming kidney function is adequate), it is probable that a disorder of gastrointestinal absorption exists. The d-xylose is used instead of glucose because several conditions may produce misleading absorption figures with glucose.

Food and drink restrictions   The patient must fast overnight before the test. Water is permitted as desired.

Procedure for collecting specimen   Laboratories vary in their specifications. Urine is voided and discarded. Then, a predetermined amount of d-xylose (usually 5 or 25 gm) is mixed with 500 ml of water and swallowed. After 1 to 2 hours, an additional 250 ml of plain water is swallowed. All urine is collected for 5 hours from the ingestion of the d-xylose. At least 150 ml of urine must be voided and collected.

Laboratory procedure   A colorimetric procedure is used.

Possible interfering materials and conditions   There may be a reduction in d-xylose excretion if the patient has taken isocarboxazid (Marplan) or phenelzine (Nardil).

Normal range   *Adults:* If the 5 gm test is used, 1.2 to 2.4 gm are normally excreted in 5 hours. *Children:* This test is not commonly performed on children.

6

Tests Performed on Feces

Although relatively few tests are done on feces, those that are performed are important to the patient whose health or life may depend on an accurate diagnosis based on such an examination. Careful collection and handling of the specimen and expert, conscientious performance of the examination are as essential as in any other test.

Blood

The discovery of blood in the feces may uncover a serious bleeding lesion of the gastrointestinal tract. Blood from a lesion in the lower colon is bright red and readily recognized. However, blood coming from the stomach or small intestine is so changed by the digestive process that it is not recognizable on inspection. Therefore, chemical tests are performed to see if there is occult blood in the feces.

Food and drink restrictions   Food restrictions vary. See next paragraph.

Procedure for collecting specimen   Sometimes, any random stool is used. At other times, since meat may also give a positive result, the physician may order the test after the patient has been on a meat-free diet for 3 days. Poultry and fish should also be omitted from such a diet.

Laboratory procedure   Several procedures are available, including tests with guaiac, benzidine, ortho-tolidine, and ortho-diamisidine. There are wide ranges in sensitivity, which are compensated for by changes in concentration. Several commercial screening tests are available.

Possible interfering materials and conditions   In some but not all of the tests, there may be a false positive reaction for occult blood in the feces if the patient has taken any of the following:

>bromides
>iodides (see Table 22)
>iron-containing medications
>meat, poultry, fish

It should also be noted that pyrvinium pamoate (Povan) stains stools red, so that there may be the appearance of frank bleeding. However, the staining is harmless.

Even on a meat-free diet, some people will normally show a positive test if their gums bleed when the teeth are brushed.

Normal range *Adults:* On a normal diet including meat, poultry, or fish, many persons will normally have positive reactions. *Children:* Same as the range for adults.

Fat Determination

This test is used to confirm the diagnosis of steatorrhea (excess fat in the stools). The steatorrhea itself may be the result of pancreatic disease, obstruction of the biliary tract, interference with intestinal absorption, conditions that block the intestinal lymphatics, or sprue.

Food and drink restrictions The patient should be on a normal diet for at least 3 days before the sample is collected.

Procedure for collecting specimen A sample of feces at least 5 gm in weight is placed in a container and sent to the laboratory. In some institutions, a 2- or 3-day sample of feces is used.

Laboratory procedure The feces sample is dried and weighed. The fat is extracted with a solvent that is subsequently evaporated. The fat that remains is then weighed.

Possible interfering materials and conditions None reported yet.

Normal range *Adults:* Between 15 and 25% of the weight of the fecal sample. *Children:* Similar to the normal range for adults.

Parasites

Examinations of feces may be performed in order to identify certain parasites or their eggs. The therapy employed usually depends on the type of parasite found, so that precise identification is important.

Food and drink restrictions   None.

Procedure for collecting specimen   The sample of feces is obtained and kept in various ways, depending on the type of parasite sought. Oily cathartics are never given. An ordinary "cold" stool is suitable for examination for ova and for amebic and similar cysts. A "warm" stool, which is kept at approximately body temperature until delivery at the laboratory, is suitable for all the previous examinations and also for trophozoites (mobile forms). A proctoscopic aspiration or scraping may be tested for trophozoites. A proctoscopic biopsy may be done to identify Schistosoma ova. Anal swabs are used to obtain material to test for pinworm eggs. All samples are taken to the laboratory at once.

Laboratory procedure   The stool samples are examined microscopically and parasites and ova identified.

Possible interfering materials and conditions   None reported yet.

Normal range   *Adults:* A large percentage of the population harbors harmless parasites such as Entamoeba coli and certain flagellates. *Children:* Same as the range for adults.

Undigested Food

The finding of large amounts of undigested food in feces specimens may indicate some abnormality of digestion.

Food and drink restrictions   None.

Procedure for collecting specimen   A stool specimen is placed in a container that is covered tightly.

Laboratory procedure   The specimen is examined macroscopically and, if requested, chemical tests for starch and fat may be performed.

Possible interfering materials and conditions   None reported yet.

Normal range   There is usually a small residue of undigested food in all feces.

Urobilinogen (Fecal)

Normally, there are considerable amounts of urobilinogen in the feces. However, in complete obstruction of the biliary tree (posthepatic), the levels of urobilinogen in the feces fall below 5 mg or 5 units per day. An increase in fecal urobilinogen suggests hemolysis.

Food and drink restrictions   None.

Procedure for collecting specimen   A stool specimen is placed in a container that is covered tightly.

Laboratory procedure   A colorimetric method is used.

Possible interfering materials and conditions   None reported yet.

Normal range   *Adults:* 75 to 350 mg urobilinogen/100 gm of stool. *Children:* This test is not commonly performed on children. The normal range is probably similar to that for adults.

7

Miscellaneous Tests

The following tests do not fall into any of the preceding categories. They measure important aspects of body function.

Basal Metabolic Rate (BMR)

This test is used much less than formerly, since more specific and accurate tests of thyroid function are now available. The BMR gives an indication of the rate at which metabolic processes take place under standard conditions. The basal metabolic rate may be elevated in such conditions as hyperthyroidism, anxiety, and infection. It may be lowered in hypothyroidism and during sedation.

Food and drink restrictions   The patient must fast for at least 10 hours before the test. Water may be taken ad lib.

Procedure for performing test   The patient, from the outset, must understand the test procedure thoroughly since any anxiety about it might change the basal metabolic rate. He should have a good night's sleep before the test. During the test the patient lies on a comfortable cot and breathes pure oxygen. The BMR machine records the amount of oxygen used per unit of time. From this, the basal metabolic rate is calculated.

Possible interfering materials and conditions   Almost any drug can affect the basal metabolic rate.

Normal range   *Adults:* −20 to +20%. *Children:* It is almost impossible to get a valid BMR measurement in children.

Biopsy

Biopsies are examinations of tissue specimens removed from patients. They may be performed on many kinds of tissue from almost any area. Biopsies may be done to help diagnose various conditions, including malignancies.

Food and drink restrictions   None, unless general anesthesia is used.

Procedure for collecting specimen   The doctor removes the specimen, using whatever technique is appropriate. A biopsy is a surgical procedure that requires the strictest aseptic precautions.

Laboratory procedure   The tissue specimen is fixed, sectioned, stained, and examined microscopically by a pathologist. In some cases, in order to save time, frozen section may be examined.

Possible interfering materials and conditions   None reported yet.

BMR   *See* Basic Metabolic Rate

Breath Alcohol

As a result of the highway accident toll, breath alcohol measurements are now being performed on automobile drivers who are suspected of being drunk or who have been involved in a serious accident. Ordinarily, a member of a police unit performs the test, and is specially trained to do so.

No one can be forced to submit to a test of breath alcohol. However, if a driver refuses to take the test, he automatically loses his license in most states. If he wishes to do so, a driver may ask that a physician draw a sample of his blood for a test (see p. 25).

The breath alcohol test has proven to be a reliable measurement of blood alcohol concentration, and there is little chance of its being in serious error despite any maneuvers of the subject.

Blood levels of alcohol under 0.05% mean that the subject is not legally considered to be under the influence of alcohol. However, even such low levels reduce driving ability significantly. Levels between 0.05% and 0.15% may or may not be considered to mean that the subject is under the influence of alcohol, depending on other evidence. Levels of 0.15% and over are considered clear evidence of being under the influence of alcohol. In many states, levels of 0.10% are now considered legal evidence that the subject is under the influence of alcohol. At levels of 0.25% and over, there is marked intoxication and beginning stupor. At about 0.40%, coma occurs, and at slightly higher levels, death can result.

Food and drink restrictions The subject must wait at least 15 minutes after his last drink of an alcoholic beverage before taking the test. This precaution is necessary to prevent a falsely high reading from traces of alcohol in the mouth. If he wishes, the subject may rinse his mouth with plain water (not mouthwash) before the test, but this is not necessary. If the subject has eaten, or drunk nonalcoholic beverages such as tea or coffee between the time of ingesting alcohol and the time of testing, the results will not be significantly affected.

Procedure for collecting specimen All instruments now on the market have disposable mouthpieces for each subject, so there need be no fear of infection. The operator gets the machine ready and, when told to do so, the subject blows into the mouthpiece. The machine utilizes the latter part of the exhaled air, which is considered alveolar air.

In some cases, the police officer may not have a testing machine available, so the subject is asked to blow into a special balloon that is then sealed and sent to a laboratory for analysis.

Laboratory procedure Special machines are used for this particular procedure. There are several on the market. Standard solutions in ampuls are used, and the ability of alcohol in the breath to change the color is measured photoelectrically. The machines are calibrated in terms of blood alcohol percentage.

Possible interfering materials and conditions Methyl alcohol (wood alcohol) and isopropyl alcohol can produce measurable levels, but they are more toxic than ethyl alcohol.

Normal range Normally there is no alcohol in the blood or breath.

Capillary Fragility *See* Tourniquet Test for Capillary Fragility

Chloride in Sweat (Screening)

This is a test for cystic fibrosis of the pancreas. It has been found that children with cystic fibrosis excrete much greater amounts of chloride in their perspiration than do normal children. Therefore, if an excessively high concentration of chloride is found in the sweat, the presumptive diagnosis becomes cystic fibrosis, and the child is treated accordingly.

Some institutions use this test in a simplified form as a routine screening test in all children. It is hoped that the test will uncover early cases that can then be treated more effectively. On the other hand, some authorities believe that the screening test should not be used, but that a chemical measurement should be made of the chloride levels in the sweat.

Food and drink restrictions   None.

Procedure for performing test   The child's hands are washed and dried. They are then kept from contact with other parts of the body for 15 minutes. After that interval, a test paper impregnated with silver chromate is moistened with distilled or tap water (*not* saline) and the patient's hand is pressed down on the paper for 4 seconds. The print is then compared to that of a normal child. Whenever chloride is present, the red silver chromate changes to white silver chloride. The imprint of the normal child's hand is indistinct, while the imprint of the hand of the child with cystic fibrosis is heavy and distinct.

Possible interfering materials and conditions   None reported yet.

Normal range   Hand print is light and indistinct.

Chloride in Sweat (Measurement)

The same general considerations apply here as to the screening test (*see* Chloride in Sweat—Screening), but the methodology is different.

Food and drink restrictions   None.

Procedure for performing test   Laboratory personnel who are experienced in doing this test should carry out the procedure, beginning with the collection of the sweat. Often, iontophoresis of a drug through the skin of the forearm is used to induce sweating. The collected sweat is then weighed and the chloride content measured as it is for serum.

Possible interfering materials and conditions None reported yet.

Normal range *Adults:* Under 60 mEq/L. *Children:* Under 40 mEq/L.

Cyanocobalamin *See* Schilling Test (Miscellaneous)

Diatrizoate Absorption Test

This test is used for early diagnosis of a perforation of the gastrointestinal tract. Its principal use is in accident cases, in which the doctor needs to know whether there has been a traumatic rupture. Diatrizoate is a substance that is not significantly absorbed by the normal gastrointestinal tract. However, it is rapidly absorbed from the peritoneal cavity and then excreted in the urine. If diatrizoate is administered to a patient without any gastrointestinal perforation, it will pass through the gut and be excreted in the feces; no significant amount will be excreted in the urine. On the other hand, if there is a gastrointestinal perforation, the diatrizoate will leak out into the peritoneal cavity, be absorbed, and be excreted in the urine.

The specific gravity of the material is high. Therefore, it tends to move down the gastrointestinal tract rapidly even if peristalsis is absent, provided the patient's position is suitable. Furthermore, since it is a radiopaque contrast medium, its location in the GI tract can readily be determined by x-ray or fluoroscopy.

The general value of this test is not yet firmly established.

Diatrizoate is available under several brand names, including Hypaque, Gastrografin, Cardiografin, and Renografin.

Food and drink restrictions When perforation is suspected, the patient should receive neither food nor water by mouth.

Procedure for performing test A urine sample is obtained from the patient, by voiding or catheterization.* The specific gravity

---

*Since the risk of gastrointestinal perforation is far greater than the risk of a urinary tract infection, there need be no hesitation about catheterizing these patients.

is measured, and 3 drops of concentrated hydrochloric acid are added slowly. No precipitate should be seen. If a precipitate is seen, the patient has probably been receiving large doses of penicillin.

The patient is then given 30 to 50 ml of diatrizoate by mouth. Moving these patients may be dangerous, since there could be other injuries. Accordingly, the nurse should not attempt to change the patient's position. This should be done by the physician or under his direct observation.

Urine samples are taken every 15 minutes for several hours. For each specimen, the specific gravity is first measured, and then 3 drops of concentrated hydrochloric acid are added.

If no precipitate forms, the chances of there being a gastrointestinal perforation are reduced.

If a thick, chalky, white precipitate forms, and was not produced in the control urine, the presumptive diagnosis is gastrointestinal perforation.

If a precipitate is noted in both control and later urines, the specific gravities are compared. If the specific gravity of the urine after administration of diatrizoate exceeds 1.040, the presumptive diagnosis is gastrointestinal perforation, since diatrizoate produces such elevations in specific gravity while other chemicals, such as penicillin, which can also cause precipitation, do not.

This test is always an emergency test, and the urine examinations should be done and reported immediately.

Possible interfering materials and conditions　Large doses of penicillin may result in a urinary precipitate after acidification, but the comparison of urine specific gravities should provide the correct diagnosis.

Normal range　Normally, no precipitate of diatrizoate will occur in the urine.

Electrocardiogram (ECG)

The electrocardiogram records the electrical potentials produced by the heart. All cells possess bioelectricity. Very sensitive instruments can pick up a difference of potential between the inside and outside of any living cell. With muscle and nerve cells, following stimulation, the cell membrane becomes permeable to certain ions, and a current flows between the inside and outside of the cell. The difference in potential travels as a wave down the cell. Our knowledge of the exact mechanisms involved is still incomplete, although most scientists believe they consist of depolarization and repolarization of the cell membrane. The electrocardiograph is a sensitive instrument, recording the changes in electrical potential of the heart that are transmitted through the limbs and chest wall. The record itself is called the *electrocardiogram*. It should be noted that only electrical potentials are measured. These electrical potentials are not directly related to force of contraction. Therefore, the electrocardiogram gives no indication as to the strength of the heart. In fact, it is possible, experimentally, to record a normal-looking electrocardiogram from a heart so weakened that no contraction whatever can be observed or recorded. The electrocardiogram is useful in diagnosing cardiac arrhythmias and in diagnosing and following the course of myocardial infarctions. Electrocardiograms are interpreted by cardiologists.

Food and drink restrictions None.

Procedure for performing test Appropriate electrodes are strapped to the patient's limbs and chest and connected to the machine that records the tracing. There are many varieties of electrocardiographs and each is operated somewhat differently from the others.

Possible interfering materials and conditions A number of drugs, including the cardiac glycosides, affect the electrocardiogram. The significance of such effects is determined by the cardiologist.

Normal range The cardiologist decides whether the tracing is normal.

Electroencephalogram (EEG)

This is a record of the electrical potentials produced by the brain cells. It may be used in the diagnosis of epilepsy and similar disorders. It is far more complex than the electrocardiogram. The electrical potentials recorded from the brain may be 100 times weaker than those recorded by the electrocardiogram, so that a much more sensitive instrument (electroencephalograph) is required to record them. Special precautions must be taken against electrical interference.

Food and drink restrictions None.

Procedure for performing test   Electrodes are fastened to the patient's scalp and connected to the machine that records the tracing.

Possible interfering materials and conditions   A number of drugs, including sedatives, may affect the EEG. The neurologist determines the significance of such effects.

Normal range   The neurologist decides whether the tracing is normal.

GA   *See* Gastric Analysis

Gastric Analysis (Tube)

This test is usually performed to determine the degree of acidity of stomach contents. Gastric contents may also be examined for enzymes, cells, and tubercle bacilli.

The tube analysis is an uncomfortable procedure for most patients, so that newer tests for gastric acidity, using various resins, have been devised (*see* Gastric Analysis, Tubeless). However, tubeless analysis is not always accurate, so that the tube analysis is still in use, although much less so than formerly.

Ordinarily, the stomach secretes hydrochloric acid to aid in digestion. In certain conditions, such as ulcers, the quantity of acid may be greater than normal, but this is not necessarily the case. In Zollinger-Ellison syndrome there is an unusually high acid secretion. In other conditions, such as pernicious anemia, gastric carcinoma, and simple achlorhydria, there may be no acid secreted. However, it is possible for patients with gastric carcinoma to have acid present in the stomach.

Gastric analysis by tube is usually contraindicated in such conditions as suspected esophageal varices, diverticula, aortic aneurysm, gastric hemorrhage, congestive heart failure, myocardial infarction, and pregnancy. It may be so uncomfortable for some patients as to be impractical. In patients with a history of asthma, urticaria, or hypertension, the histamine augmentation part of the test is contraindicated.

In many cases, the patient having a gastric analysis will require increased care and attention from the nursing staff for the duration of the test. If the augmented histamine procedure is used, the patient must be observed *continuously* until the test is completed. Severe reactions, including loss of consciousness, may result from the injection of the histamine or histamine producer. Epinephrine solution and a syringe and needle should be ready on a tray in case they are needed to counteract a severe reaction.

Food and drink restrictions   These vary from laboratory to laboratory. Often, the patient receives nothing by mouth after supper on the night before the test.

Procedure for collecting the specimen   The general procedure should be explained to the patient when the test is ordered so as to minimize apprehension. A physician should perform the intubation. Either the oral or nasal route is used, depending on the physician's experience and on the patient's gag reflex.

The tube is chilled with ice to help reduce nausea, and is lubricated. Often, its position is adjusted by the doctor using a fluoroscope.

The gastric contents are aspirated by syringe. Sometimes intermittent and sometimes continual withdrawal are used.

The augmented histamine test is sometimes added, since histamine is a potent stimulant of stomach acid secretion. After the basal stomach contents have been aspirated, the physician injects a measured amount of histamine or Histalog. Usually, an antihistamine is given about 30 minutes before the histamine. It counteracts most of the unpleasant side effects but does not significantly interfere with acid secretion.

Laboratory procedure   The amount of hydrochloric acid in each sample is measured by titration.

Possible interfering materials and conditions   None reported yet.

Normal range   *Adults:* About 8% of healthy persons have no gastric acid. The earlier distinctions between free and total acidity are no longer of significance. The normal range is about 5 to 40 mEq HCl/hr after histamine stimulation. *Children:* This test is not usually performed on children.

Gastric Analysis (Tubeless)

This method of determining the presence of stomach acid does not require the passing of a tube into the esophagus and is more comfortable for the patient. It is based on the fact that free hydrochloric acid will displace certain materials from combination with other substances. The earlier tubeless analyses were performed with quininium resin indicator. More recently, an azure indicator dye has been used.

In general, this method is not suitable for exact quantitative analysis but gives the essential information needed in many cases, i.e., whether free acid is present in the stomach. Since false negative reactions sometimes occur, a negative report is not diagnostic of achlorhydria unless confirmed by standard gastric analysis. The tubeless method can save most patients from the discomfort of intubation.

Food and drink restrictions   No food is taken after midnight, but water is permitted as desired.

Procedure for collecting specimen   In the morning, the first urine specimen is discarded. The patient is then given a glass of water with 500 mg of caffeine sodium benzoate. After one hour he urinates, and the urine specimen is saved as a control. He then swallows the blue granules of the dye in one-half glass of water. After an additional 2 hours he urinates, and the urine is sent to the laboratory. The urine may be blue or green for several days after. This has no significance.

Laboratory procedure   Both urine specimens are diluted, and aliquots are compared to standards.

Possible interfering materials and conditions   In patients who have had such operations as subtotal gastrectomy, gastroenterostomy, pyloroplasty, both false negative and false positive results may occur. In patients with malabsorption syndrome, severe diarrhea, pyloric obstruction, severe liver disease, severe kidney disease, severe dehydration, or urinary retention, the results of this test may be misleading.

The diagnex blue level may be falsely elevated if the patient has taken any of the following within the preceding 2 days:

aluminum	methylene blue
antacid medications	nicotinic acid
barium	Pomalin
calcium	potassium, large amounts
Cremomycin	quinacrine (Atabrine)
Donnagel	quinidine
iron	quinine
kaolin	riboflavin
Kaopectate	sodium (large amounts)
magnesium	vitamin B capsules

In addition, phenazopyridine (Table 17), which colors the urine orange, may make it impossible to obtain any reading.

Normal range   A blue color equal to or more than 0.6 mg standard indicates the presence of hydrochloric acid in the stomach.

Gastrointestinal Perforation   *See* Diatrizoate Absorption

Microscopic Tests for Malignant Cells (Papanicolaou Smear)

In many areas of the body, malignant (cancer) cells separate from tumors and may be identified microscopically. This may make possible the diagnosis of malignancy early enough for satisfactory treatment or even complete cure. Such tests are most commonly performed on the female genital tract but are also of value in other areas. Other specimens include: bronchial, esophageal, rectal, and colonic washings; duodenal drainage; gastric and nipple secretions; pleural, peritoneal, and pericardial exudates; prostate smears; sputum; and urine.

Food and drink restrictions   None.

Procedure for collecting specimen   The physician collects the specimen. If it consists of a washing, drainage, exudate, aspiration fluid, or urine, it is mixed with equal parts of 95% alcohol and sent to the laboratory. If it consists of a smear or a secretion, it is smeared on a glass slide that is then immersed in a solution containing equal parts of 95% alcohol and ether *before the smear can dry*. Sputum is collected in 70% alcohol. Other types of fixing solutions are also available and may be used for some specimens.

Laboratory procedure   The fluid specimens are concentrated by centrifugation and smeared. All smears are stained and examined microscopically.

Normal range   Normally, no malignant cells are found.

Mucin Clot Test

This is a rough test of the amount of hyaluronate in the synovial (joint) fluid. If a "poor" mucin clot is produced, there is a strong likelihood of inflammation in the joint.

Food and drink restrictions   None.

Procedure for collecting specimen The specimen is collected *only* by a physician, using aseptic technique. The exact procedure used depends on the joint involved, and should be in accord with orthopedic surgical standards.

Laboratory procedure The synovial fluid is added to an acetic acid solution and the nature of the clot observed.

Possible interfering materials and conditions None reported yet.

Normal range *Adults:* The clot is described as "good" or "fair." *Children:* This test is not usually done on children.

Papanicolaou Smear *See* Microscopic Tests for Malignant Cells

Pregnancy Tests *See* Chapter 5

Radioiodine Uptake

This test is used in the diagnosis of thyroid conditions. It is based on the fact that the radioactive isotope of iodine, I^{131}, is taken up by the thyroid in the same manner as ordinary iodine. The breakdown of I^{131} to more stable elements results in the release of gamma rays, which can be detected and counted by a scintillation counter held near the patient's neck. The degree of radioactivity is a measure of the degree of iodine uptake. Uptake below normal ranges suggests hypothyroidism; uptake above normal ranges suggests hyper-thyroidism. The amount of radioactivity involved is too small to harm the patient, and much too small to be a hazard to anyone else. This test should be distinguished from the use of radioiodine in *therapy*, where much larger amounts are used.

Food and drink restrictions None.

Procedure for performing test No special preparation is necessary. The patient's past history must be checked for any excess iodine consumption, which would give misleading test results. If the patient has taken any of the drugs listed in Table 22 within a 30-day period, that information should be given to the radiology laboratory at once. If the patient has had x-ray studies of the gallbladder, ureters, bronchi, fallopian tubes, heart, or other organs in which iodinated contrast media were used, that information should be noted, even if many years have elapsed. If the patient has eaten large amounts of sea food in the previous 2 weeks, that fact too should be noted. When necessary, the patient may be assured that the amount of radioactivity involved is too small to do any harm. Furthermore, it can be pointed out that I^{131} has a short half-life (8 days), so that it will disappear rapidly. The patient can continue normal food and water intake. A capsule containing the radioactive iodine is swallowed by the patient. After exactly 6 or 24 hours, the amount of radioactivity coming from the thyroid gland is measured in the radiology laboratory, using a scintillation counter. Sometimes, 24-hour urines are also collected and measured for radioactivity. After the test is completed, the patient may be given some Lugol's solution, or other medication containing regular iodine. This will displace most of the remaining radioactive iodine from the body.

Possible interfering materials and conditions If the patient has received, during the preceding 30 days, any of the iodine-containing drugs listed in Table 22, there may be a misleading depression of radioiodine uptake. Some breads in which iodides are used as dough conditioners may also cause lower readings. In addition, other drugs that can depress the radioiodine uptake, listed by official (generic) name, include:

ACTH
antihistamines
butazolidin
chlordiazepoxide
chlortetracycline
cortisone (see Table 20)
diazepam
methimazole
methylthiouracil
nitrates
para-aminosalicylic acid
penicillin
phenothiazines (see Table 25)
phenylbutazone
sulfonamides
testosterone
thiopental
thiouracil
thyroglobulin
thyroid, dessicated
thyronine
thyroxine

A misleading elevation of the radioiodine uptake may be produced by estrogens (see Table 21).

Since there are so many materials that can give misleading

results in this test, other, more specific tests of thyroid functions are beginning to replace it (*see* T3 Uptake, T4, TSH, and Thyroid Antibodies, Chapter 3, Tests Performed on Blood).

Normal range   *Adults:* This depends to some extent on the iodine content of the food eaten. As more iodine is added to prepared foods, normal values tend to decrease. The normal range is now considered to be 5 to 15% uptake at 6 hours and 12 to 35% uptake at 24 hours. *Children:* Similar to adult, when the I^{131} is given in a dose proportional to size.

Ropes Test   *See* Mucin Clot Test

Rumple-Leede Test   *See* Tourniquet Test for Capillary Fragility

Schilling Test

This is a test for pernicious anemia and related conditions. Patients with pernicious anemia and certain other disorders cannot absorb cyanocobalamin (Vitamin B_{12}) properly. Therefore, when radioactive cyanocobalamin is given orally, and followed by intramuscular nonradioactive cyanocobalamin, the excretion of radioactive cyanocobalamin in the urine is less than normal. The test is usually given in stages. If the first stage shows a normal urinary excretion of cyanocobalamin, pernicious anemia is probably not present, and the test is terminated. But if the first stage shows a lower than normal urinary excretion of radioactive cyanocobalamin, a second, and possibly a third stage of testing may be needed to rule out conditions other than pernicious anemia that can cause decreased gastrointestinal absorption of cyanocobalamin.

Stage 1

Food and drink restrictions   The patient must fast for at least 12 hours before the test and during the test until he receives the injection of nonradioactive cyanocobalamin. Water is permitted. No laxatives may be used.

Procedure for collecting specimen   The patient voids and the urine is discarded. Then 0.5 microcuries of radioactive cyanocobalamin are swallowed. From this point on, all urine is collected for 24 hours and stored. No special preservatives or refrigeration are needed for the urine, but complete collection is vital.

Two hours after taking the radioactive cyanocobalamin orally, the patient receives 1 mg of nonradioactive cyanocobalamin by intramuscular or intravenous injection. (Some authorities recommend that this be given 30 minutes rather than 2 hours after the oral administration. Check with the laboratory as to the method preferred.)

The patient may eat after the injection of nonradioactive cyanocobalamin.

If Stage 1 of this test shows a lower than normal excretion of radioactive cyanocobalamin in the urine (under 7%), Stage 2 is performed.

Stage 2

It is advisable to wait 5 days after Stage 1 before performing Stage 2, although in some institutions the wait may be shorter.

Food and drink restrictions   The patient must fast for at least 12 hours before the test and during the test until he receives the injection of nonradioactive cyanocobalamin. Water is permitted. No laxatives may be used.

Procedure for collecting specimen   The patient voids and the urine is discarded. Then, 0.5 microcuries of radioactive cyanocobalamin are swallowed, plus 60 milligrams of intrinsic factor from pigs. From this point on, all urine is collected for 24 hours and stored. No special preservatives or refrigeration are needed for the urine, but complete collection is vital.

Two hours after taking the radioactive cyanocobalamin orally, the patient receives 1 mg of nonradioactive cyanocobalamin by intramuscular or intravenous injection. (Some authorities recommend that this be given 30 minutes rather than 2 hours after the oral administration. Check with the laboratory as to the method preferred.)

The patient may eat after the injection of nonradioactive cyanocobalamin.

If Stage 2 of this test shows an excretion of over 7% of the radioactivity in 24 hours, and if Stage 1 showed less than 7%, the probable diagnosis is pernicious anemia. If, however, both Stages 1 and 2 show a 24-hour excretion of radioactivity under 7%, Stage 3 is performed.

Stage 3

Stage 3 is carried out to discover whether an alteration in the bacteria of the intestine is interfering with absorption of cyanocobalamin and producing signs and symptoms similar to pernicious anemia. Stage 3 requires 11 days for completion.

Food and drink restrictions   For the first 9½ days of this stage of the test, there are no restrictions. But the patient must fast for at least 12 hours before the administration of the cyanocobalamin and continue to fast during the test until he receives the injection of nonradioactive cyanocobalamin. Water is permitted. No laxatives may be used.

Procedure for collecting specimen   For 10 days, the patient receives tetracycline, 250 mg four times daily by mouth (to reduce the bacteria in the gastrointestinal tract). At the end of this period, the procedure described for Stage 1 is repeated.

If the excretion of radioactivity after Stages 1 and 2 had been less than 7%, and if after Stage 3 it is more than 7%, the probable diagnosis is bacterial interference with cyanocobalamin absorption.

Laboratory procedure   The radioactivity of an aliquot of the urine is measured in a scintillation counter.

Possible interfering materials and conditions   Therapeutic doses of cyanocobalamin given in the 3 days preceding the test may interfere with interpretation of the results.

Kidney disease may cause a deceptively low excretion of the radioactivity during the test period. In such cases, a prolonged testing period may be required.

Normal range   *Adults:* Normally, the 24-hour excretion of radioactive cyanocobalamin in Stage 1 is greater than 7% of the amount ingested. *Children:* This test is not commonly performed on children, and the normal range is not definitely established.

Sputum Smears for Eosinophiles and Elastic Fibers

The sputum contains eosinophiles in cases of allergic asthma, but not in ''cardiac'' asthma. Finding eosinophiles may, therefore, aid in the differential diagnosis between these two conditions. If elastic fibers are found in the smear, there is probably a destructive lesion of the walls of the alveoli or bronchioles, such as tuberculosis with cavitation, malignancy, or lung abscess.

Food and drink restrictions None.

Procedure for collecting specimen Sputum is collected in a container that is then covered. In some institutions the sputum is smeared on 2 slides in the patient's room. Elsewhere, the smearing is done in the laboratory.

Laboratory procedure The slides are stained and examined microscopically for eosinophiles and elastic fibers.

Possible interfering materials and conditions None reported yet.

Normal range *Adults:* Normally there are very few, if any, eosinophiles or elastic fibers in the sputum. *Children:* Similar to the range for adults.

Thorn Test

This is an indirect test of adrenal function named after its originator. It has been replaced by the more direct serum cortisol measurement.

Tourniquet Test for Capillary Fragility

This test measures the ability of the capillaries to remain intact under stress. Increased capillary fragility may be found in many types of systemic vascular abnormalities, including scurvy, thrombocytopenic purpura, and purpura accompanying severe infections.

Procedure for performing test The physician inflates a blood pressure cuff on the patient's arm to a point midway between diastolic and systolic pressures. The pressure is maintained for 10 minutes. Any petechiae (small hemorrhages under the skin) render the test positive. Sometimes counts of petechiae per unit of area may also be reported.

Possible interfering materials and conditions None reported yet.

Normal range *Adults:* Some people will normally have a positive reaction, particularly those with red hair. *Children:* This test is not commonly performed on children.

Xylose *See* Chapter 5

8

Normal Values in Infants and Children

In infants and children, the normal ranges for many tests differ considerably from those of adults. Some of the more striking differences are summarized in this chapter.

Blood

At birth, the infant usually has a higher hemoglobin content than the adult. The average is about 17 gm/100 ml, but higher concentrations are normal. This high level falls rapidly. At the age of 2 months it is about 14 gm/100 ml and at about 3 months it reaches a low point of about 11 gm/100 ml. Thereafter, the hemoglobin content tends to rise very slowly, reaching about 13 gm/100 ml at the age of 2 years.

The red blood cells follow a similar pattern.

The white blood cells (leucocytes) are very numerous at birth. They average 20,000 per cu mm of blood, but counts as high as 35,000 per cu mm are normal. This is about 4 times the adult level. The leucocyte count falls gradually, but remains higher than the adult level for at least the first 2 years of life. Accordingly, an elevated leucocyte count in a young infant has little or no diagnostic significance.

The infant normally has some degree of icterus with an elevated serum bilirubin from the second to the seventh day of life. This results from two factors—a considerable degree of destruction of the red blood cells and immaturity of the liver.

On the other hand, an excessive degree of icterus or visible icterus within 24 hours of birth may denote a serious condition, such as erythroblastosis fetalis, which requires prompt, efficient therapy.

In newborn infants a low fasting blood glucose, about 50

mg/100 ml or sometimes even lower, is common. This rises gradually, reaching 75 mg/100 ml in the small child.

The total cholesterol in newborn infants is quite low, ranging from 80 to 165 mg/100 ml of blood. However, this level rises until, in most children, it reaches 200 to 300 mg/100 ml. This is higher than usual adult levels. It may not represent a strictly physiologic change. There is a strong likelihood that the high serum cholesterol levels in American children result from their high intake of dairy products after the age of weaning.

The alkaline phosphatase levels are high, up to 20 Bodansky units, because of the formation of new bone cells.

During the first few days of life the level of blood urea nitrogen may be as high as 40 mg/100 ml of blood. However, it rapidly falls to the adult level.

In the newborn the blood potassium level may be as high as 7 mEq/L. It, too, soon drops to adult levels.

Cerebrospinal Fluid

In the newborn the glucose levels in the cerebrospinal fluid may normally be as low as 35 mg/100 ml. This, of course, is correlated with the low blood glucose levels. As the blood glucose levels rise, so do the CSF levels.

Urine

Albuminuria is a common, almost universal, finding in infants during the first week or two of life. In older children it may or may not indicate the presence of disease.

Infants and children under 8 years of age normally excrete practically no 17-ketosteroids. At the age of 8, excretion increases gradually, reaching adult levels at about age 18. Increased levels in infants and young children may result from adrenal hyperplasia.

9

Units of Measurement Used in Clinical Laboratory Procedures

A *gram* (gm) is a standard unit of weight or mass.

A *milligram* (mg, mgm) is 1/1000 of a gram.

A *microgram (mcg, microgm, mcgm, gamma) is* 1/1,000,000 of a gram.

A *nanogram* (ng) is 1/1,000,000,000 of a gram.

A *milligram percent* is a milligram per 100 cubic centimeters or per 100 grams.

A *cubic centimeter* (cc) is a unit of volume equal to a cube 1 centimeter in each dimension. It is equivalent to a milliliter (1/1000 of a liter) for practical purposes.

A *cubic millimeter* (cu mm) is a unit of volume equal to a cube 1 millimeter in each dimension. It is equivalent to 1/1000 of a cubic centimeter for practical purposes.

A *liter* (L) is a unit of liquid measurement. It is equivalent to 1000 cubic centimeters, or about 1 quart.

A *volume percent* is a measurement of the amount of gas dissolved in a liquid. For example, when 10 cc of gas is dissolved in 100 cc of fluid, the concentration can be expressed as 10 volumes percent.

A *mol* is the number of grams equal to the number that expresses the molecular weight of the substance. Since sodium, for example, has a weight of 23, a mol of sodium is 23 grams.

A *molar* solution is a mol of a substance dissolved in enough fluid to make 1 liter of solution. Thus a molar solution of sodium has 23 grams of sodium per liter.

A *millimol* is 1/1000 of a mol. A millimol of sodium is 23 milligrams.

A *millimolar* solution is a millimol of a substance dissolved in enough fluid to make 1 liter of solution. A millimolar solution of sodium contains 23 milligrams of sodium per liter.

An *equivalent* is a mol divided by a valence. An equivalent of sodium is 23/1 or 23 grams. An equivalent of calcium (weight 40, valence 2) is 40/2 or 20 grams.

A *milliequivalent* (mEq) is 1/1000 of an equivalent. A milliequivalent of sodium is 23 milligrams and a milliequivalent of calcium is 20 milligrams.

A *unit* is an arbitrary measurement used when no other means of measurement is satisfactory. Units are usually based on a particular bioassay technique. The unit in one kind of test bears no relationship to the unit in another kind of test.

Part Two

Tables and Reference Data

Table 1. Tests of Blood Function and for Blood Disorders

Test	Performed on
Albumin	Blood
Bilirubin, partition	Blood
Bilirubin, total	Blood
Bleeding time	Capillaries of skin
Blood counts	Blood
Blood culture	Blood
Blood types	Blood
Calcium	Blood
Clotting time	Blood
CO_2 combining power	Blood
Coombs' direct	Blood
Coombs' indirect	Blood
Fibrinogen	Blood
Globulin	Blood
Glucose-6-phosphate dehydrogenase	Red blood cells
Haptoglobin	Blood
Hematocrit	Blood
Hemoglobin	Blood
Hemoglobin electrophoresis	Red blood cells
Iron	Blood
Iron binding capacity	Blood
Magnesium	Blood
Malaria film	Blood
Methemoglobin	Blood
Partial thromboplastin time	Blood
PCO_2	Blood
pH	Blood
Plasma electrophoresis for gammopathies	Blood
Platelet count	Blood
PO_2 (arterial)	Blood
Porphyrins	Urine

Table 1. Tests of Blood Function and for Blood Disorders (cont'd.)

Test	Performed on
Potassium	Blood
Protein	Blood
Prothrombin time	Blood
Red cell fragility	Blood
Reticulocyte count	Blood
Schilling	Urine
Sedimentation rate	Blood
Sickle cell test	Blood
Sodium	Blood
Sulfhemoglobin	Blood
Tourniquet test for capillary fragility	Capillaries of skin of arm
Urinary blood	Urine

Table 2. Test of Liver Function and for Liver Disorders

Test	Performed on
Ammonia	Blood
Bilirubin, partition	Blood
Bilirubin, total	Blood
Bromsulphalein retention (BSP)	Blood
Cephalin flocculation	Blood
Cholesterol	Blood
Fecal urobilin	Feces
Glucose	Blood
Glucose tolerance	Blood and urine
Phosphatase, alkaline	Blood
Prothrombin time	Blood
Serum transaminase	Blood
Thymol turbidity	Blood
Urinary bile and bilirubin	Urine
Urobilinogen	Urine

Table 3. Tests of Kidney Function and for Kidney Disorders

Test	Performed on
Albumin (qualitative and quantitative) in urine	Urine
Calcium	Blood
Chlorides	Blood
CO_2 combining power	Blood
Concentration and dilution	Urine
Creatinine	Blood and urine
Creatinine clearance	Urine and blood
Microscopic tests of urinary sediment	Urine
Phenolsufonphthalein (PSP)	Urine
Phosphorus	Blood
Potassium	Blood
Sodium	Blood
Specific gravity	Urine
Urea nitrogen	Blood

Table 4. Tests of Metabolic Function and for Metabolic Disorders

Test	Performed on
Amino acids	Urine
Ammonia	Blood
Ascorbic acid	Blood
Ascorbic acid tolerance	Blood
Ascorbic acid tolerance	Urine
Basal metabolic rate (BMR)	Patient
Calcium	Blood
Carbon dioxide	Blood
Folic acid	Blood
Glucose	Blood
Glucose tolerance	Blood and urine
Guthrie	Blood
Homogentisic acid	Urine
Ketone bodies (blood)	Blood
Ketone bodies (urine)	Blood
Lipid fractions	Blood
Lipoprotein analysis	Blood
Osmolality, serum	Blood
pH	Blood
Phenylketonuria	Urine
Radioiodine uptake	Patient
Sugar, qualitative and quantitative	Urine
Triglycerides	Blood
Uric acid	Blood

Table 5. Tests for Infections, Microorganisms, and Resistance to Microorganisms

Test	Performed on
Agglutination	Blood
Antistreptolysin O titer	Blood
Australia antigen assay	Blood
Bacterial count, urine	Urine
Blood culture	Blood
Cold agglutinins	Blood
C-reactive protein	Blood
Fluorescent antibody	Many substances
Fluorescent treponemal antibody absorption	Blood
Heterophile antibody	Blood
Malaria film	Blood
Miscellaneous fluid cultures	Body fluids
Mono-Diff	Blood
Nose and throat culture	Nose and throat secretions
Parasites	Stool
Rapid plasma reagin	Blood
Rubella antibody	Blood
Sedimentation rate	Blood
Serological tests	Blood and spinal fluid
Special tests	Spinal fluid
Spinal fluid chlorides	Spinal fluid
Spinal fluid culture	Spinal fluid
Spinal fluid protein	Spinal fluid
Spinal fluid sugar	Spinal fluid
Sputum culture and smear	Sputum
Stool culture	Stool
Urine culture	Urine
White cell differential count	Blood
Wound culture	Wound exudates

Table 6. Tests for Malignancy

Test	Type of Malignancy	Performed on
Aschheim-Zondek, quantitative	Teratoma	Urine
Bence Jones protein	Bone tumors	Urine
Carcinoembryonic antigen assay		Blood
Catecholamines	Pheochromocytoma	Urine
5-Hydroxyindoleacetic acid	Carcinoid	Urine
Melanin	Melanomas	Urine
Microscopic tests	All	Various fluids
Papanicolaou	All	Various fluids
Phosphatase, acid	Prostate carcinoma	Blood
Phosphatase, alkaline	Bone tumors	Blood
Vanilmandelic acid	Pheochromocytoma	Urine

Table 7. Tests of Endocrine Glands and Their Functions

Test	Gland	Performed on
Amylase	Pancreas	Blood
Amylase, urine	Pancreas	Urine
Calcium	Parathyroid	Blood
Calcium (Sulkowitch)	Parathyroid	Urine
Cortisol	Adrenal cortex	Blood
Glucose (sugar)	Pancreas	Blood and urine
Glucose tolerance	Pancreas	Blood and urine
17-Hydroxycorticosteroids	Adrenal cortex	Urine
17-Ketogenic steroids	Adrenal cortex	Urine
17-Ketosteroid excretion	Adrenal cortex	Urine
Lipase	Pancreas	Blood
Phosphorus	Parathyroid	Blood
Potassium	Adrenal cortex	Blood
Protein-bound iodine (PBI)	Thyroid	Blood
Radioiodine uptake	Thyroid	Patient
Sodium	Adrenal cortex	Blood
Thyroid antibodies	Thyroid	Blood
Thyroid stimulating hormone	Thyroid	Blood
Thyroxine	Thyroid	Blood
T3 resin uptake	Thyroid	Blood

Table 8. Tests for Poisoning

Test	Performed on
Alcohol	Blood and breath
Aminolevulinic acid	Urine
Barbiturates	Blood
Bromides	Blood
Carbon monoxide	Blood
Lead	Blood and urine
Methemoglobin	Blood
Porphyrins	Urine
Salicylates	Blood
Sulfhemoglobin	Blood

Table 9. Tests for Myocardial Infarction

Test	Performed on
Creatine phosphokinase	Blood
Electrocardiogram	Patient
Heat-stable lactic dehydrogenase	Blood
Lactic dehydrogenase	Blood
Lactic dehydrogenase isoenzymes	Blood
Myoglobin, quantitative	Urine
Transaminase (serum)	Blood

Table 10. Tests Performed on Venous Blood

Test	ml of blood	Color of stopper	Normal range Adults	Normal range Children
Agglutination	5	Red	See test	See test
Albumin	6	Red	3.2 - 5.6 gm/100 ml (serum albumin)	3.2 - 5.6 gm/100 ml
			1.3 - 3.5 gm/100 ml (serum globulin)	2.2 - 3.3 gm/100 ml
			6 - 8 gm/100 ml (total serum protein)	Varies with age (see test)
Alcohol	5 to 10	Green, red, or gray, depending on laboratory	Negative	Negative
Aldolase	3	Red	Depends on method	Depends on method
Ammonia	5	Green	Under 75 - 100 mcg/100 ml	Under 75 - 100 mcg/100 ml
Amylase	5	Red	80 - 150 U (Somogyi)	Not usually performed
Antistreptolysin O titer	5	Red	Under 160 Todd U/100 ml	Varies with age (see test)
Antinuclear antibodies	2	Red	Negative	Negative
Ascorbic acid	5	Gray	0.6 - 1.6 mg/100 ml	0.6 - 1.6 mg/100 ml

208

Table 10. Tests Performed on Venous Blood (cont'd.)

Test	ml of blood	Color of stopper	Normal range Adults	Children
Ascorbic acid tolerance	5	Gray	1.6 mg/100 ml or more	Not usually performed
Australia antigen assay	Done by blood bank		Negative	Negative
Barbiturate	5 to 10	Green or red, depending on laboratory	Negative	Negative
Bilirubin, partition	5	Red	See test	See test
Bilirubin, total	5	Red	0.1 - 1.0 mg/100 ml	0.2 - 0.8 mg/100 ml
Blood types	5	Red	Any	Any
Bromides	5	Green	Negative	Negative
Bromsulphalein	7	Red	under 0.4 mg/100 ml (under 5% retention)	Not usually performed
Calcium	5	Red	4.5 - 5.7 mEq/L	Varies with age (see test)
Carbon dioxide	Full tube	Varies	See test	See test
Carbon monoxide	7	Lavender	See test	See test
Carcinoembryonic antigen assay	Full tube	Lavender	Under 2.5 ng/ml	Not usually performed
Carotene	4 to 10	Red	40 - 300 mcg/100 ml	Not usually performed

Table 10. Tests Performed on Venous Blood (cont'd.)

Test	ml of blood	Color of stopper	Normal range	
			Adults	Children
Cephalin flocculation	5	Red	Neg. to 1+	Not usually performed
Ceruloplasmin	3	Red	20 - 35 mg/100 ml	See test
Chlorides	5	Red	95 - 106 mEq/L	95 - 106 mEq/L
Cholesterol	5	Red	See test	See test
Clotting time	4 × 1	None	See test	See test
CO_2 combining power	7	Green	24 - 35 mEq/L	No longer usually performed
Cold agglutinins	7	Red	Titer under 1:16	Titer under 1:16
Coombs' direct	2	Red	Negative	Negative
Coombs' indirect	5	Red	Negative	Negative
Cortisol	5 to 10	Varies	See test	Not usually performed
C-reactive protein	5	Red	Negative	Negative
Creatine phosphokinase	5	Red	See test	See test
Creatinine	5	Red	0.6 - 1.3 mg/100 ml	0.4 - 0.5 mg/100 ml
Cryoglobulins	3 to 10	Red	Negative	Negative
Culture	Varies	Yellow in most laboratories	Negative	Negative

Table 10. Tests Performed on Venous Blood (cont'd.)

Test	ml of blood	Color of stopper	Normal range Adults	Children
Digitoxin and digoxin	5	Red	See test	See test
Diphenylhydantoin	5	Red	See test	See test
Fibrinogen	Full	Blue or orange	200 - 600 mg/100 ml	200 - 600 mg/100 ml
Fluorescent treponemal antibody absorption	5	Red	Negative	Negative
Folic acid	7	Red	See test	Not usually performed
Glucose	5	Gray	See test	See test
Glucose-6-phosphate dehydrogenase	See test	Varies	Positive	Positive
Glucose tolerance	Varies	Red or gray	See test	See test
Haptoglobin	5	Red	100 - 200 mg/100 ml	See test
Heat-stable lactic dehydrogenase	3 to 5	Red	Below 115 units	Not usually performed
Hematocrit	Full	Lavender	35 - 50%	See test
Hemoglobin electrophoresis	Full	Lavender	Only hemoglobin A	See test
Heterophile antibody	5	Red	Under 1:28	Under 1:28

Table 10. Tests Performed on Venous Blood (cont'd.)

Test	ml of blood	Color of stopper	Normal range	
			Adults	Children
Immunoglobulins	5 to 10	Red	See test	See test
Iron	10	Red	60 - 200 mcg/100 ml	55 - 185 mcg/100 ml
Iron-binding capacity	10	Red	250 - 425 mcg/100 ml	Same as for adults
Ketone bodies	3	Red	2 - 4 mcg/100 ml	Similar to that for adults
Lactic dehydrogenase	5	Red	See test	See test
Lactic dehydrogenase isoenzymes	5	Red	See test	Not usually performed
Lead	Full	Green or brown	0 - 80 mcg/100 ml	Same as for adults
Lipase	up to 10	Red	Under 1.5 U/ml	Not usually performed
Lipid fractions	10	Red	See test	See test
Lipoprotein analysis	4	Red	See test	See test
Lithium	5	Red	See test	Not usually performed
Lupus erythematosus cell test	Varies	Varies	Negative	Negative
Magnesium	3	Red	1.8 - 3 mcg/100 ml	2.0 - 2.6 mcg/100 ml

212

Table 10. Tests Performed on Venous Blood (cont'd.)

Test	ml of blood	Color of stopper	Normal range		
			Adults		Children
Malaria film	At least ½ tube	Lavender	Negative		Negative
Methemoglobin	Full	Green or lavender	Negative		Negative
Mono-Diff	2	Red	Negative		Negative
Osmolality	5 to 10	Red	275 - 295 milliosmols/kg water		270 - 285 milliosmols/kg water
Partial thromboplastin time	Full	Blue	See test		See test
Partial pressure of CO_2	Full	Green	35 - 40 mm mercury		35 - 43 mm mercury
pH	5	Green	7.35 - 7.45		7.38 - 7.42
Phosphatase, acid	5	Red	See test		Not usually performed
Phosphatase, alkaline	5	Red	See test		See test
Phosphorus	5	Red	1.8 - 2.6 mEq/L		See test
PO_2	Full	Green	See test		See test
Potassium	5	Red	3.8 - 5 mEq/L		3.8 - 5 mEq/L
Protein-bound iodine	8	Red	4 - 8 mcg/100 ml		4 - 8 mcg/100 ml
Prothrombin time	Full	Blue	See test		See test

Table 10. Tests Performed on Venous Blood (cont'd.)

Test	ml of blood	Color of stopper	Normal range	
			Adults	Children
Rapid plasma reagin	5	Red	Negative	Negative
Red cell fragility	Full	Lavender	See test	See test
Rheumatoid arthritis test	5	Red	See test	See test
Rubella antibody	3	Red	See test	See test
Salicylates	5	Green	See test	See test
Sedimentation rate	4	Lavender	See test	See test
Serological tests	5	Red	Negative	Negative
Serum glutamic oxaloacetic transaminase	5	Red	See test	See test
Serum glutamic pyruvic transaminase	5	Red	See test	See test
Sickle cell test	3	Lavender	See test	See test
Sodium	5	Red	136 - 142 mEq/L	136 - 142 mEq/L
Special microorganisms	10	Red	Negative	Negative
Sulfhemoglobin	5	Green	Negative	Negative
Sulfonamide level	5	Green	See test	See test
Thymol turbidity	5	Red	Under 5 units	Not usually performed

Table 10. Tests Performed on Venous Blood (cont'd.)

Test	ml of blood	Color of stopper	Normal range Adults	Normal range Children
Thyroid antibodies	5	Red	See test	Not usually performed
Thyroid stimulating hormone	5	Red	Up to 0.2 mU/ml	Not usually performed
Thyroxine	5	Red	See test	See test
T3 resin uptake	5	Red	25 - 35%	Not established
Triglycerides	5	Red	See test	Not established
Urea nitrogen	5	Red	9 - 20 mg/100 ml	9- 20 mg/100 ml
Uric acid	5	Red	See test	See test

Table 11. Tests Performed on Capillary Blood

Test	Normal range Adult	Children
Bleeding time	1 - 6 min	1 - 6 min
differential (see white cell differential count)		
Erythrocyte (see red cell count)		
Guthrie	Not usually performed	Negative
Hemoglobin	12 - 18 gm/100 ml	Varies with age (see test)
Leucocyte (see white cell count)		
Platelet count	150,000 - 400,000/cu mm	After first week, similar to that for adults
Red cell count	4 - 6 million/cu mm	Varies with age (see test)
Reticulocyte count	0.1 - 1.5/100 red cells	Probably similar to that for adults
White cell count	4,000 - 11,000/cu mm	Varies with age (see test)
White cell differential count	Neutrophils 54 - 62% Eosinophils 1 - 3% Basophils 0 - 1% Lymphocytes 25 - 33% Monocytes 0 - 9%	Varies with age (see test)

Table 12. Tests Performed on Cerebrospinal Fluid

Test	ml of fluid	Normal range Adults	Children
Cell count (leukocyte)	1 to 2	0 - 8 cells/cu mm	0 - 8 cells/cu mm
Chlorides	2	118 - 133 mEq/L	120 - 128 mEq/L
Culture	2	Negative	Negative
Protein	2	15 - 45 mg/100 ml	15 - 45 mg/100 ml
Serology	7	Negative	Negative
Sugar	2	45 - 75 mg/100 ml	35 - 75 mg/100 ml

Table 13. Tests Performed on Urine

Test	Urine sample	Normal range
Albumin	Random	None, or small amounts
Amino acids	Random or 24 hr	*Adult*—300 - 650 mg/24 hr
		Children—see test
Aminolevulinic acid	Random or 24 hr	See test
Amylase	Timed sample	Under 270 units/hr
Ascorbic acid tolerance	5- or 6-hr sample	Oral—10% of administered amount
		Intravenous—30 - 40% of administered amount
Bacterial count	Clean sample	Under 10,000/ml
Bence Jones protein	Random	None
Bile and bilirubin	Random	None
Blood	Random	A few red cells (see test)
Calcium (Sulkowitch)	Random	A fine white precipitate
Catecholamines	24 hr	Depends on laboratory
Chlorides, quantitative	24 hr	See test
Concentration and dilution	Several at specified intervals (see test)	Concentration—specific gravity over 1.025
		Dilution 1.003 - 1.005
Creatinine	24 hr	See test
Creatinine clearance	24 hr	100 - 140 ml/min
Estriol	24 hr	20 mg/24 hr or higher after 35th week
Homogentisic acid	Random	None
5-Hydroxyindoleacetic acid	24 hr	2 - 10 mg/24 hr
17-Hydroxy corticosteroids	24 hr	4 - 14 mg/24 hr
Immunologic test for pregnancy	Random or morning	See test
Ketone bodies	Random	None

Table 13. Tests Performed on Urine (cont'd.)

Test	Urine sample	Normal range
17-Ketogenic steroids	24 hr	See test
17-Ketosteroids	24 hr	See test
Lead	24 hr	Under 100 mcg/24 hr
Melanin	Random	None
Microscopic	Random	See Test
Morphine	Special	None
Myoglobin (general)	Random	None
Myoglobin, quantitative	Random	None
pH	Random	4.8 - 8.0
Phenolsulfonphthalein (PSP)	Random	Elimination of 10 - 50% in first 15 min
Phenylhetonuria	Random	None
Porphobilinogen (qualitative)	During or immediately after pain	None
Porphobilinogen (quantitative)	24 hr	Under 2 mg/24 hr
Porphyrins	24 hr	Minute quantity to none
Specific gravity	Random	1.001 - 1.035
Sugar, qualitative	Random	None
Sugar, quantitative	24 hr	116 - 656 mg/24 hr
Urobilinogen	2 hr or random	Not over 2.5 mg/24 hr
Vanilmandelic acid	24 hr	Not over 7.5 mg/24 hr
d-Xylose tolerance (oral)	5 hr total, minimum 150 ml	For 5 gm test, 1.2 - 2.4 gm/5 hr

Table 14. Tests Performed on Feces

Test	Fecal specimen	Normal range
Blood (guaiac or benzidine)	Random, or following meat-free diet, as ordered	May be positive on random specimen
Fat	Random	15 to 25% of weight of dried sample
Parasites	As ordered (see test)	Harmless parasites such as E. coli and flagellates are normal
Undigested food	Random	Small amounts
Urobilin	Random	Large amounts

Table 15. Miscellaneous Tests

Test	Specimen	Normal range
Basal metabolic rate (BMR)	Patient	−20 to +20%
Breath alcohol	Expired air	None
Chloride in sweat	Hand (see test)	Light, indistinct hand print
Diatrizoate excretion	Patient & urine	None
Electrocardiogram (ECG)	Patient	Interpretation by cardiologist
Electroencephalogram (EEG)	Patient	Interpretation by neurologist
Gastric analysis	Gastric fluid	Depends on stimulus (see test)
Gastric analysis, tubeless	2-hr urine specimen (see test)	More than 25 microgm quinine, or blue color not less than 0.6 mg azure A standard
Microscopic tests for malignant cells	Various body fluids	None
Radioiodine uptake	Patient	See test
Sputum smears	Sputum	Few eosinophiles or elastic fibers
Tourniquet for capillary fragility	Capillaries of skin of arm	Usually negative

Table 16. Partial List of Drugs and Mixtures Containing Androgens

(Asterisk indicates either official or common name)

Adroyd	*Fluoxymesterone	*Norethandrolone
Anadrol	Formatrix	Ora-testryl
Anavar	Geriatric preparations	Oreton
Android	(several)	Os-cal-mone
Deca-Durabolin	Gevrestin	*Oxandrolone
Deladumone	Gevrine	*Oxymetholone
Delatestryl	Gynetone	Perandren
Deop-testadiol	Halodrin	Premarin with
Depo-Testosterone	Halotestin	methyl testosterone
Dianabol	Hovizyme	Ritonic
*Dromostanolone	Mediatric	*Stanozolol
Dumogran	Metandren	*Testosterone
Dumone	*Methandriol	Tylosterone
Durabolin	*Methandrostenolone	Ultandren
Eldec	*Methyltestosterone	Winstrol
*Ethylestrenol	Nandrolone	Zeste M. T.
*Femandren	Nilevar	

Table 17. Partial List of Drugs and Mixtures Containing Azo Dyes

(Asterisk indicates either official or common name)

Azo Gantanol	Azotrex	Pyridium
Azo Gantrisin	Buren	Suladyne
Azolate	Dolonil	Thiosulfil A
Azo-Mandelamine	Donnasep	Uremide
Azophene	Mallophene	Urobiotic
Azo-Sulfurine	*Phenazopyridine	

Table 18. Partial List of Drugs and Mixtures Containing Barbiturates

(Asterisk indicates either official or common name)

*Allylbarbituric acid	Amytal	Bellergal
Alurate	*Aprobarbital	Bentyl/pb
Amesec	*Barbital	Brevital
*Amobarbital	Belladenal	*Butabarbital

Table 18. Partial List of Drugs and Mixtures Containing Barbiturates (cont'd.)

*Butallylonal	Ilocalm	Quadamine
*Butethal	Ipral	Quadrinal
Butibel	Lotusate	Sandoptal
Butigetic	Luasmin	*Secobarbital
Butiserpine	Luminal	Secodrin
Butisol	Mebaral	Seconal
Carbrital	Mebroin	Seconesin
Chardonna	Medomin	Sibena
Cholan HMB	*Methitural	Solfoserpine
Codempiral	*Methohexital	Solfoton
*Cyclobarbital	Nebralin	Sombulex
Dainite	Nembudeine	Spasticol S. A.
Daprisal	Nembudonna	Stental
Deltasmyl	Nembugesic	Surital
Delvinal	Nembutal	Synirin
Desbutal	Neconal	*Talbutal
Dexamyl	Neocholan	TCS Tablets
Dialog	Neraval	Tedral
Donnatal	Nidar	Tepalate
Donnazyme	*Pentobarbital	Tetrasule-S
Empiral	Pentothal	*Thiamylal
Eskabarb	Percobarb	*Thiopental
Eskaphen	Pernoston	Tuinal
Ethalyl	Phanodorn	Valpin-Pb
Evipal	Phenaphen	Veronal
Fiorinal	*Phenobarbital	*Vinbarbital
Halabar	Plexonal	Zamitol
*Heptabarbital	*Probarbital	
*Hexobarbital	Prolaire	

Table 19. Partial List of Drugs and Mixtures Containing Chloral Hydrate

Aquachloral	Kessodrate	Somnos
Beta-Chlor	Loryl	Triclos (enzymatic
En-Chlor	Noctagetic	action reduces
Fello-Sed	Noctec	to same active
Felsules	Rectules	metabolite as
		chloral hydrate)

Table 20. Partial List of Drugs and Mixtures Containing Cortisone or Its Derivatives

(Asterisk indicates either official or common name)

Acne-Cort-Dome	Delta-Cortef	Lida-Mantle
Alflorone	Delta-Dome	Lidex
Alphadrol	Deltasmyl	Lipo-Adrenal Cortex
Anusol	Deltasone	Locorten
Aquacort	Deronil	Magnacort
Aristocort	Deltra	Medrol
Aristoderm	Deltrasone	*Methylprednisolone
Aristogesic	Depo-Medrol	Meticortetone
Aristomin	Derma Medicone-HC	Meticorten
Ataraxoid	Deronil	Meti-Derm
Aural acute	*Desoxycorticosterone	Metimyd
Benisone	Dexameth	Metreton
*Betamethasone	*Dexamethasone	Mycolog
Betapar	Domeform	Neo-Aristocort
Blephamide	Dronactin	Neo-Aristoderm
Caldecort	Es-A-Cort	Neo-Cortef
Carbo-Cort	F-Cortef	Neo-Decadron
Celestone	Fernisolone-B	Neo-Delta-Cortef
Chymar	Florinef	Neo-Deltef
Collosul HC	*Fludrocortisone	Neo-Cort-Dome
Conjunctilone	Fluonid	Neo-Hydeltrasol
Cordran	*Fluorometholone	Neo-Medrol
Cort-Acne	Formtone	Neo-Oxylone
Cor-Tar-Quin	Gammacorten	Neosone
Cortate	Haldrone	Neo-Synalar
Cort-Dome	Hebcort	Optef
Cortef	Hexaderm	Otobione
Cortifan	Hexadrol	Oxylone
*Cortisol	Hist-A-Cort	Pabalate-HC
*Cortisone	Hycortole	Pabirin
Cortogen	Hydeltra	Pantho-F
Cortone	Hydeltrasol	Paracort
Cortril	*Hydrocortamate	Paracortol
Decadron	*Hydrocortisone	*Paramethasone
Decagesic	Hydrocortone	Percorten
Decaspray	Hytone	Predne-Dome
Decortin	Kenacort	Prednefrin
Decosterone	Kenalog	*Prednisolone
Delenar	Ledaform-HC	*Prednisone

222

Table 20. Partial List of Drugs and Mixtures Containing Cortisone or Its Derivatives (cont'd.)

Protef	Somacort	Triamel-HC
Rectal Medicone-HC	Sterane	Vio-Fernisone
Respihaler Decadron	Sterazolidin	Vioform-
Respihaler Pro	Sterne	Hydrocortisone
Decadron	Sterolone	Vio-Hydrosone
Salcort	Synalar	Vio-Hydrosone
Servisone	Tarcortin	Vytone
Sigmagen	Tenda Cream	Ze-Tar-Quin
Solu-Cortef	Terra-Cortril	Zetone
Solu-Medrol	*Triamcinolone	

Table 21. Partial List of Drugs and Mixtures Containing Estrogens

(Asterisk indicates either official or common name)

*Benzestrol	Estradurin	Milprem
*Chlorotrianisene	*Estriol	Ogen
Clusivol	*Estrone	Ovocylin
Cylogesterin	Evex	PMB
Deladumone	Femandren	Premarin
Delestrogen	Formatrix	Progynon
Deluteval	Furestrol	Provest
Depo-Estradiol	Gerilets	Quinette
Depo-Testadiol	Gevrestin	SK Estrogens
Dicorvin	Gyneton	Sulestrex
*Diethylstilbesterol	Halodrin	Tace
*Dinestrol	*Hexestrol	Theelin
Duosterone	Hormonin	Ultrogen
*Equilenin	Hovizyme	Urestrin
*Equilin	Lutocylol	Vallestril
Estinyl	Menest	Zeste
*Estradiol	*Methallenestril	

Table 22. Partial List of Drugs and Mixtures Containing Iodine

(Asterisk indicates either official or common name)

Part A—Therapeutic Agents

Amend's solution
Arocalcin
Bronchoid, Jr.
Calathesin
Calcidrine
Ceradine
Cher-Iomine
Child's Drikof
Creodide
Dainite KI
Darbid
Di-Iodo Tyrosine
*Dough conditioners (some)
Elixophyllin KI
Endoarsan
Entero-Vioform
Entodon
Feosol powders & tablets
Floraquin
Iocapral
Iocylate
Iod-Ethamine
Iodex
Iodized Petrogen
Iodo-Ichthyol

Iosalex ointment
Isopropamide Iodide
Isuprel Compound Elixir
Itrumil
Limodin
Lipoiodine
*Lugol's solution
Milpath
Mudrane
*Nail polish
Organidin
Oridine
Pediacof
*Potassium iodide
Quadrinal
Quin-O-Creme
*Sodium iodide
Tamponets
Theokin
Theo-organidin
Thyractin
*Tincture of iodine
Tuss-organidin
Vioform

Part B—Radiographic Contrast Media

Name (Asterisk indicates either official or common name)	Period during which all iodine determinations including protein-bound and radioiodine uptake will probably be meaningless
*Acetrizoate	2 weeks
Cardiografin	2 weeks
*Chloriodized oil	1 to 5 years
Cholografin	2 to 6 months
Conray	2 to 6 months
Diodrast	2 to 6 months
*Diatrizoate	2 weeks
Dionosil	2 to 6 months
Diprotrizoate	2 weeks

Table 22. Part B—Radiographic Contrast Media (cont'd)

Ethiodol	1 to 5 years
Gastrografin	2 weeks
Hypaque	2 weeks
*Iodipamide	2 to 6 months
*Iodized oil	1 to 5 years
*Iodoalphionic acid	2 to 6 months
Iodochloral	1 to 5 years
*Iopanoic acid	2 to 6 months
*Iophendylate	1 to 5 years
*Iophenoxic acid	2 to 6 months
*Iodopyracet	2 to 6 months
*Iothalamate	1 to 5 years
*Ipodate	2 to 6 months
Lipiodol	1 to 5 years
Mediopaque	2 weeks
*Meglumine iothalamate	2 to 6 months
Miokon	2 weeks
Neo-ipax	2 weeks
Oragrafin	2 to 6 months
Pantopaque	1 to 5 years
Priodax	2 to 6 months
*Propyliodone	2 to 6 months
Renographin	2 weeks
Salpix	2 to 6 months
Skiodan	2 to 6 months
Telepaque	2 to 6 months
Teridax	2 to 6 months
Thixokon	2 weeks
Urokon	2 weeks
Visciodol	1 to 5 years

Table 23. Partial List of Drugs and Mixtures Containing Meprobamate

Appetrol	Equanitrate	Miltown
Bamadex	Kessobamate	Miltrate
Cyclex	Meprospan	Pathibamate
Deprol	Meprotabs	PMB
Equagesic	Milpath	Prozine
Equanil	Milprem	SK Bamate

Table 24. Partial List of Drugs and Mixtures Containing Oxytetracycline

(Asterisk indicates either official or common name)

Oxlopar	Terra-Cortril	Terrastatin
Oxy-Tetrachel	Terramycin	Urobiotic
*Oxytetracycline		

Table 25. Partial List of Drugs and Mixtures Containing Phenothiazine Derivatives

(Asterisk indicates either official or common name)

*Acetylpromazine	*Methoxypromazine	Serentil
*Acetophenazine	Mornidine	Sparine
*Carphenazine	Neozine	Stelazine
Chlorphenergan	Notensil	Tacaryl
*Chlorpromazine	Pacatal	Temaril
*Chlorpromethazine	Parsidol	Tentone
Combid	Pernitil	*Thiethylperazine
Compazine	*Perphenazine	*Thioperazine
Coplexen	Phenergan	*Thiopropazate
Dartal	*Pipamazine	*Thioridazine
*Diethazine	*Prochlorperazine	Thoradex
Diparcol	Proketazine	Thorazine
Eskatrol	Prolixin	Tindal
*Ethapropazine	Promapar	Torecan
*Fluphenazine	*Promazine	*Trifluoperazine
Largon	*Promethazine	*Triflupromazine
Mellaril	*Propiomazine	Trilafon
*Mepazine	Prozine	*Trimeprazine
Mepergan	*Pyrathiazine	Veractil
*Methdilazine	Pyrrolazote	Vesprin
*Methotrimeprazine	Quide	Vontil

226

Table 26. Partial List of Drugs and Mixtures Containing Reserpine

Butiserpazide	Metamine	Salutensin
Butiserpine	Metatensin	Sandril
Diupres	Naquival	Ser-Ap-Es
Diutensin	Penite	Serpasil
Eskaserp	Rau-sed	Serpatilin
Hydromox R	Regroton	Solfoserpine
Hydropres	Renese-R	Unitensen
Iphyllin	Reserpoid	

Table 27. Partial List of Drugs and Mixtures Containing Salicylates

(Asterisk indicates either official or common name)

*Acetylsalicylic acid	Equagesic
Anacin	Excedrin
Arlcaps	Fiorinal
A.S.A.	Measurin
Ascodeen	Medaprin
*Aspirin	*Methyl salicylate
Bufferin	Monacet Compound
Cama	Nembu-Gesic
Codempiral	Pabalate
Coldene	Pabirin
Cordex	Percobarb
Coricidin	Percodan
Corilin	Phenaphen
Daprisal	Pyrroxate
Darvon Compound	Robaxisal
Darvo-Tran	Salcedrox
Dasin	Salcort
Decagesic	*Salicylate, sodium
Delenar	Sigmagen
Ecotrin	Stero-darvon/ASA
Edrisal	Synalgos
Empiral	Thephorin-AC
Empirin	Trancogesic
Emprazil	Zactirin Compound

Selected References

Periodicals

Allen, R. J., and Wilson, J. L. Urinary phenylpyruvic acid in phenylketonuria. *J.A.M.A., 188*:720, 1964.

Alvarez, W. C. A great need for evaluating laboratory tests. *Modern Medicine,* April 1, 1958, p. 10.

Aring, C. D. An occupation for adults. *Arch. Int. Med., 116*:164, 1965.

Astin, T. W. Systemic reaction to bromsulphthalein. *Brit. Med. J., 2*:408, 1965.

Baer, D. M., and Krause, R. B. Spurious laboratory values resulting from simulated mailing conditions. *Am. J. Clin. Path., 50*:111-119, 1968.

Barnett, R. N., Civin, W. H., and Schoen, I. Multiphasic screening by laboratory tests—an overview of the problem. *Am. J. Clin. Path., 54*:483-492, 1970.

Beeson, P. B. The case against the catheter. *Am. J. Med., 24*:1, 1958.

Behringer, B. R., and Stephenson, H. E., Jr. The diatrizoate precipitation test for intestinal perforation. *Surg., Gynec. & Obstet., 129*:475-482, 1969.

Berry, H. K., Sutherland, B., Guest, G. R., and Warkany, J. Simple method for detection of phenylketonuria. *J.A.M.A., 167*:2189, 1958.

Betson, C. Blood gases. *Amer. J. Nursing, 68*:1010-1012, 1968.

Blum, N. I., Mayoral, L. G., and Kalser, M. H. Augmented gastric analysis—a word of caution. *J.A.M.A., 191*:339, 1965.

Briller, A. Important uses of electrocardiography. *Amer. J. Nursing, 55*:1378, 1955.

Bronson, W. R., DeVita, V. T., Carbone, P. P., and Cotlove, E. Pseudohyperkalemia due to release of potassium from white blood cells during clotting. *New Eng. J. Med., 274*:369, 1966.

Brown, P. A. The cost of clinical laboratory testing. *J.A.M.A., 229*:1350, 1974.

Brown, W. J. Acquired syphilis: Drugs and blood tests. *Amer. J. Nursing, 72*:939, 1972.

Caraway, W. T. Chemical and diagnostic specificity of laboratory tests. *Am. J. Clin. Path., 37*:445, 1962.

Castleman, B. Normal laboratory values. *New Eng. J. Med., 262*:84, 1960.

Charles, D., Van Leeuwen, L., and Turner, J. H. Significance of cornified cells in the vaginal smear of postmenopausal women. *Am. J. Obstet. Gynec., 94*:527, 1966.

Clark, M. B. Studies based on errors observed in the use of anticoagulants in blood chemistry determinations. *Am. J. Med, Technol., 17*:190, 1951.

Clarke, T. H., and Laipply, T. C. The use and abuse of laboratory tests in surgery. *Surg. Clin. N. America, 44*:3, 1964.

Clayton, E. M., Altschuler, J., and Bove, J. R. Penicillin antibody as a use of positive direct antiglobulin tests. *Amer. J. Clin. Path., 44*:648, 1965.

Cohen, L. Serum enzyme determinations: their reliability and value. *Med. Clin. N. America, 53*:115-135, 1969.

Cranswick, E. H., Cooper, T. B., and Simpson, G. M. Two-year follow-up study of protein-bound iodine elevation in patients receiving perphenazine. *Am. J. Psychiat., 122*:300, 1965.

Cripps, G. W., Martiney, D. R., Gillism, R. A., and Caldwell, T. J. Significance of drug-altered laboratory test values. *Amer. J. Hosp. Pharm., 30*:603, 1973.

Croft, J. D., Jr., et al. Coombs'-test positivity induced by drugs. *Ann. Int. Med., 68*:176-186, 1968.

David, R. R., Alexander, D. S., and Wilkins, L. Placental transfer of an organic radiopaque medium resulting in a prolonged elevation of the protein-bound iodine. *J. Pediat., 59*:223-226, 1961.

Dawborn, J. K., and Plunkett, P. J. The collection and assessment of mid-stream urine samples in the diagnosis of urinary tract infection in women. *Med. J. Australia,* April 13, 1963, p. 540.

Deu, S. D. Testing for glycosuria. *Amer. J. Nursing, 70*:1513, 1970.

Didisheim, P. Tests of blood coagulation and hemostasis. *J A.M.A., 196*:33, 1966.

Dlouhy, A., Erickson, M. B., Sr., Nedlicka, B., Imburgia, F., Ipavec, J., and Kiewlich, S. What patients want to know about their diagnostic tests. *Nursing Outlook, 11*:265, 1963.

Duhme, D. W., Greenblatt, D. J., and Koch-Weser, J. Reduction of digitoxin toxicity associated with measurement of serum levels. *Ann. Int. Med., 80*:516, 1974.

Elevebach, L. R., Guillier, C. L., and Keating, F. R., Jr. Health, normality, and the ghost of Gauss. *J.A.M.A., 211*:69-75, 1970.

Finlay, J. M., Hogarth, J., and Wightman, K. J. R. A clinical evaluation of the D-xylose tolerance test. *Ann. Int. Med., 61*:411, 1964.

Fisher, A. B., Levy, R. P., and Price, W. Gold—an occult cause of low serum protein-bound iodine. *New Eng. J. Med., 273*:812, 1965.

Fogel, B. J., Sanders, R. W., Fife, E. H., and Anderson, R. I. The serodiagnosis of early syphilis. How to utilize the newer laboratory tests. *Clin. Ped., 4*:447, 1965.

Foster, M. A. Teaching blood groups and reactions. *Nursing Outlook,* Feb. 1966, p. 49.

Foulk, W. T., and Fleisher, G. A. The effects of opiates on the activity of serum transaminase. *Proc. Staff Meet. Mayo Clin., 32*:405, 1957.

Gault, M. H., and Dossetor, J. B. Editorial: The place of phenolsulfonphthalein (PSP) in the measurement of renal function. *American Heart J., 75*:723-727, 1968.

Goldstein, A., and Brown, B. W., Jr. Urine testing schedules in methadone maintenance treatment of heroin addiction. *J.A.M.A., 211*:315, 1970.

Goldthwait, J. C., Butler, C. F., and Stillman, J. S. The diagnosis of gout. *New Eng. J. Med., 259*:1095, 1958.

Grant, S. D., Foshman, P. H., and DiRaimondo, V. C. Suppression of 17-hydroxycorticosteroids in plasma and urine by single and divided doses of triamcinolone. *New Eng. J. Med., 273*:1115, 1965.

Guze, L. B., and Beeson, P. B. Observations on the reliability and safety of bladder catheterization for bacteriologic study of the urine. *New Eng. J. Med., 255*:474, 1956.

Hartney, J. B. The role of the clinical laboratory in the community hospital. *Med. Clin. N. America, 53*:11-23, 1969.

Haunz, E. A. The role of urine testing in diabetes detection. *Amer. J. Nursing, 64*:102, 1964.

Hayner, N. S., *et al.* Carbohydrate tolerance and diabetes in a total community, Tecumseh, Mich. *Diabetes, 14*:413, 1965.

Heath, H., Lee, R. B., Dimond, R. C., and Wartofshy, L. Conjugated estrogen therapy and tests of thyroid function. *Ann. Int. Med., 81*:351, 1974.

Jackson, G. G., and Greeble, H. G. Pathogenesis of urine infection. *Arch. Int. Med., 100*:692, 1957.

Journal of the American Medical Association (Editorial). The shrinking specificity of the transaminase determination. *J.A.M.A., 191*:101, 1965.

Journal of the American Medical Association (Editorial). Urinary phenylpyruvic acid in phenylketonuria. *J.A.M.A., 188*:748, 1964.

Kraus, S. J., Haserick, J. R., and Lantz, M. A. Atypical FTA-ABS test flourescence in lupus erythematosus patients. *J.A.M.A., 211*:2140-2141, 1970.

Kushner, D. S. Phenolsulfonphthalein excretion test. *J.A.M.A., 195*:1078, 1966.

Linton, K. B., and Gillespie, W. A. Collection of urine from women for bacteriological examination. *J. Clin. Path. 22*:376-380, 1969.

London, W. T., Vought, R. L., and Brown, F. A. Bread—a dietary source of large quantities of iodine, *New Eng. J. Med., 273*:381, 1965.

Luddecke, H. F. Basal metabolic rate, protein-bound iodine and radioactive iodine uptake: a comparative study. *Ann. Int. Med., 49*:305, 1958.

Mainwaring, C. Clean voided specimens for mass screening. *Amer. J. Nursing, 63*:96, 1963.

Mallin, S. R., and Gambescia, J. M. A fatal reaction to sulfobromophthalein. *J.A.M.A., 174*:1858, 1960.

Marks, V., and Shackcloth, P. Diagnostic pregnancy tests in patients treated with tranquilizers. *Brit. Med. J., 1*:517, 1966.

Martin, M. M. New trends in diabetes detection. *Amer. J. Nursing, 63*:101, 1963.

McBay, A. J. Carbon monoxide poisoning. *New Eng. J. Med., 272*:252, 1965.

McCraw, J. B., Mcleod, R. A., and Stephenson, H. E., Jr. A urine precipitation test for intestinal perforation. *Arch. Surg., 91*:248, 1965.

Merrett, D. A., and Sanford, J. P. Sterile voided urine culture. *J. Lab. Clin. Med.,* *52*:463, 1958.

Meyer, R. R. Effect of iopanoic acid on the sulfobromophthalein test. *J.A.M.A., 194*:343, 1965.

Moertel, C. G., Beahrs, O. H., Woolner, L. B., and Tyce, G. M. Maligant carcinoid syndrome associated with noncarcinoid tumors. *New Eng. J. Med., 273*:244, 1965.

Myer, G. G. Disseminated intravascular coagulation. *Amer. J. Nursing, 73*:2092, 1973.

O'Leary, L. Electro-encephalography. *Amer. J. Nursing, 55*:1238, 1955.

Oltman, J. E., and Friedman, S. Further report on protein-bound iodine in patients receiving perphenazine. *Amer. J. Psychiat., 121*:176, 1964.

Peters, T., Jr., and Davis, J. S. Serum heat-stable lactate dehydrogenase in the diagnosis of myocardial infarction. *J.A.M.A., 209*:1186-1190, 1969.

Pfeffer, R. B., Stephenson, H. E., Jr., and Hinton, J. W. The effect of morphine, demerol and codeine on serum amylase values in man. *Gastroenterology, 23*:482, 1953.

Pierce, J. M., Jr., Ruzumna, R., and Segar, R. Standardization of the phenolsulfonphthalein excretion test in clinical practice. *J.A.M.A., 175*:711, 1961.

Reagan, J. W. Cytological studies. *Amer. J. Nursing, 58*:1693, 1958.

Reznikoff, P., and Engle, R. L. The physician, the laboratory and the patient. *GP, 26*:82, 1962.

Rivin, A. U. False endocrine test results due to drugs. *Calif. Med., 101*:283, 1964.

Russe, H. P. The use and abuse of laboratory tests. *Med. Clin. N. America, 53*:223-231, 1969.

Sapira, J. D., Klaniecki, T., and Ratkin, G. Non-pheochromocytoma. *J.A.M.A., 212*:2243-2245, 1970.

Scardino, J. Lithium in affective disorders. *N.Y. State J. Med., 70*:638-642, 1970.

Scheiner, L. B., Rosenberg, B., Marathe, V. V., and Pech, C. Differences in serum digoxin concentrations between outpatients and inpatients: an effect of compliance? *Clin. Pharmacol. and Ther., 15*:234, 1975.

Schneider, E. M. Venous abnormalities following intravenous sodium sulfobromophthalein administration. *J.A.M.A., 194*:339, 1965.

Shapiro, R., and Man, E. B. Iophenoxic acid and serum-bound iodine values, *J.A.M.A., 173*:1352, 1960.

Silberstein, E. B. The Schilling test. *J.A.M.A., 208*:2325-2326, 1969.

Smith, A. M., Theirer, J. A., and Huang, S. H. Serum enzymes in myocardial infarction. *Amer. J. Nursing, 73*:277, 1973.

Spangler, A. S., Jackson, J. H., Fiurmara, N. J., and Warthin, T. A. Syphilis with a negative blood test reaction. *J.A.M.A., 189*:87, 1964.

Stephenson, H. E., Jr., McCraw, J., and McLeod, R. Early diagnosis of abdominal trauma. *Missouri Med., 63*:267, 1966.

Stewart, M. J. Testing home tests for cervical cancer. *Amer. J. Nursing, 65*:75, 1965.

Switzer, S. The clean voided urine culture in surveying populations for urinary tract infection. *J. Lab. Clin. Med., 55*:557, 1960.

Vandervelde, E. M. et al. User's guide to some new tests for hepatitis B antigen. *Lancet, 2*:1066, 1974.

Wilkinson, J. H. Clinical significance of enzyme activity measurements. *Clin. Chem., 16*:882-890, 1970.

Wirth, W. A., and Thompson, R. L. The effect of various conditions and substances on the results of laboratory procedures. *Am. J. Clin. Path., 43*:579, 1965.

York, P. S., Landes, R. R., and Seay, L. S. Coombs' positive reactions associated with cephaloridine therapy. *J.A.M.A., 206*:1086, 1968.

Books

Bennington, J. L., Fouty, R. A., and Hougie, C. *Laboratory Diagnosis.* London: Macmillan, 1970.

Davidsohn, I., and Henry, J. B. *Clinical Diagnosis by Laboratory Methods,* 15th ed. Philadelphia: W. B. Saunders, 1974.

Frankel, S., Reitman, S., and Sonnenwirth, A. C. *Gradwohl's Clinical Laboratory Methods and Diagnosis,* 6th ed. St. Louis: C. V. Mosby, 1963.

Henry, R. J., Cannon, D. C., and Winkelman, J. W. *Clinical Chemistry: Principles and Technics,* 2d ed. New York: Harper and Row, 1974.

Wallach, J. *Interpretation of Diagnostic Tests,* 2d ed. Boston: Little, Brown & Co., 1974.

Widmann, F. K. *Clinical Interpretation of Laboratory Tests,* 7th ed. Philadelphia: F. A. Davis, 1973.

Index